THE MANAGEMENT HANDBOOK
FOR PRIMARY CARE

The Management Handbook for Primary Care

Essential management skills for Primary Care professionals

Edited by Tim Swanwick

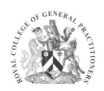

The Royal College of General Practitioners was founded in 1952 with this object:

> "To encourage foster and maintain the highest possible standards in general practice and for that purpose to take or join with others in taking steps consistent with the charitable nature of that object which may assist towards the same."

Among its responsibilities under its Royal Charter the College is entitled to:

> "Diffuse information on all matters affecting general practice and issue such publications as may assist the object of the College."

British Library Cataloguing-in-Publication Data
A catalogue record for this book is available from the British Library

© Royal College of General Practitioners, 2004
Published by the Royal College of General Practitioners 2004
14 Princes Gate
Hyde Park
London
SW7 1PU

Cover and text designed and typeset by discript.com, London
Printed by Bell & Bain Ltd, Glasgow
Indexed by Carol Ball

ISBN 0 85084 288 3

Contents

Preface

This is a handbook of management skills for general practitioners and other Primary Care workers who find themselves, perhaps unexpectedly, in management positions. The book is not a manual of practice management or a vade mecum for practice managers, rather it focuses on useful techniques and methods for the day-to-day management of people, projects, and organisations. This is a skills-based book and, after reading each chapter, you should have the confidence to 'have-a-go', or at least have developed an insight as to how things might go better next time!

The handbook is orientated towards Primary Care rather than General Practice, although many of the chapters are written specifically with the general practitioner in mind. This, in a sense, encapsulates the College's dilemma of maintaining General Practice at the centre of its activity whilst inviting other allied professions in to collaborate on the development of Primary Care. Issues such as appraisal, organisational development, change management, and team working are relevant to us all, and I hope that despite its publication under the aegis of the Royal College of General Practitioners – indeed, many of the contributors are practising GPs – colleagues from all the disciplines working in Primary Care will find this book useful.

Similarly, the handbook has been written with the whole of the UK in mind, and I must ask for the understanding of colleagues in Scotland, Wales, and Northern Ireland who will need to translate some of the Anglo-centric organisational terminology – of which Primary Care Trust is the most frequent example – into their own national context.

Tim Swanwick
London, October 2003

Acknowledgements

This book was conceived during the 2002 RCGP Leadership Programme and would not be here had it not been for one of the programme's learning sets. Thanks then to Jill Edwards, Julia Oxenbury, and Clare Gerada, who have also contributed magnificently to the book, Penny Trafford for her unfailing support, and Stephen Kelly who also identified the funds to make it all happen. Royalties from the sale of copies of this book will be donated to the RCGP Leadership Programme.

Grateful thanks also to Monica White and Deepti Jayawardena Wilkinson for their assistance in putting it all together.

Tim Swanwick
London, October 2003

About the authors

The editor

Tim Swanwick

Tim has a broad range of experience in General Practice education and educational management. Currently a Director of Postgraduate General Practice Education at the London Deanery, Tim is also a member of the panel of examiners of the Royal College of General Practitioners, sits on the editorial board of *Education for Primary Care*, and writes widely on all aspects of General Practice education and training. Recent publications include *The General Practice Journey* (2003) and *The Study Guide for General Practice Training* (2003).

The contributors

Tim Swanwick
Director of Postgraduate General Practice Education
London Deanery

Antony Americano
Head of Human Resources and Central Services
London Department of Postgraduate Medical and Dental Education
University of London

Julia Whiteman
Deputy Director of Postgraduate General Practice Education
London Deanery

Julia Oxenbury
Associate Director of Postgraduate General Practice Education
Wessex Deanery

Fraser Macfarlane
Lecturer in Health Care Management
School of Management, University of Surrey

Andrew Wilson
Associate Director of Postgraduate General Practice Education for London and Eastern Deaneries, Convenor of the written paper of the MRCGP examination

John Schofield
Quality Medical Consultant
Qual-Med Ltd

David Claridge
Freelance Consultant in Co-operation and Negotiation

Jan Pearcey
Primary Care Education Lead
Hillingdon Primary Care Trust

Jill Edwards
Associate Director of Postgraduate General Practice Education
Oxford Deanery

David Haslam
Chairman of Council
Royal College of General Practitioners

Roger Neighbour
President
Royal College of General Practitioners

Helen Alpin
Chairman
Professional Executive Committee for East Leeds Primary Care Trust

Clare Gerada
Director of Primary Care
National Clinical Governance Support Team

Neil Jackson
Dean of Postgraduate General Practice Education
London Deanery

Chapter 1

The Management of Primary Care

Tim Swanwick

 KEY MESSAGES
- Primary Care in the National Health Service is a complex system requiring expert and sympathetic management.
- General practitioners and allied professionals are ideally placed to manage Primary Care owing to their transferable skills, insider knowledge, the peculiar nature of professional organisations, and their proven positive impact on change.
- Management is an activity and not a profession.

Management – there's a lot of it about

Kate has been with her three-partner practice for eight years and runs the financial aspects of the surgery together with her practice manager. She developed an interest in quality and 18 months ago was persuaded to take on the clinical governance lead for her Primary Care Group. Following 'devolution day' on April 1 2002, Kate was elected to join the Board of her local Primary Care Trust (PCT). It has been a steep learning curve and due to a colleague's long-term illness, she has been standing in as PCT Chief Executive for the last three months. Kate is now responsible for a budget of £50M, a staff of 900, and the commissioning of secondary care for a population of 120,000.

In today's National Health Service (NHS), doctors, nurses, and other health care professionals are increasingly required to assume management responsibility. Professional cynics, and indeed cynical professionals, would argue that clinicians' time would be better spent doing what they were trained for; that is, concentrating on the improvement of individual patient outcomes rather than on the management of the systems in which those endeavours are undertaken. But health care is complex, probably now more so than ever, involving a mutable interaction between people, their surroundings, and the resources available to them.[1] Complex systems require effective management and as Edwards[2] highlights, '... there is a mounting body of evidence that badly managed organisations fail patients, frustrate staff, deliver poor quality care, and cannot adapt to the rapidly changing environment in which they operate'.

Not only is the world changing rapidly, the pace of change is accelerating. Of course, as Berwick is careful to point out,[3] not all change is improvement. All improvement, however, is change and to effectively bring about change requires expert management. Improving or changing health care for the better depends on changing systems, not simply on working harder within them; system improvement requires influencing the behaviour of others and influencing others is management.

The new Primary Care-led NHS is designed to bring decision making nearer to the patient.[4] It is inevitable then that management decisions will increasingly involve practitioners of all disciplines working within Primary Care. New organisational structures have institutionalised this approach, the archetype of which is the Primary Care Trust (PCT) with its heavy reliance on a professionally led executive committee. Meanwhile, the 2003 GP contract is set to reward a range of organisational practice attributes with quality payments.

Management skills are valued then, even at practice level, indeed 'professionally expected', as the following excerpt from *Good Medical Practice for General Practitioners*[5] serves to illustrate.

The excellent GP

- has effective systems for communication within the practice
- holds regular meetings with members of the practice team
- knows how to contact individual members of the team outside meetings
- understands the health needs of the local population and tries to ensure that the Primary Care team has the skills to meet those needs
- aims to develop an organisation that offers personal and professional development opportunities to its staff

Outside the practice, GPs and other practitioners may assume a wide variety of management roles, sometimes voluntarily, occasionally by default, but almost always, as in Kate's case, without preparation or training. Examples of just some of the management roles currently undertaken by practitioners, both directly and indirectly associated with patient care, are shown in Box 1.1.

So there's a lot of it about – management, that is. What's more, there is in today's NHS a pressing need for management competence, expertise, and therefore training, a need that has been acknowledged officially in two recent public inquiries.[6,7] As Ian Kennedy summarises in *Learning from Bristol*:

Box 1.1 **Management roles for Primary Care practitioners.**
- PCT Chief Executive
- Director of Primary Care (PCT/Health Authority)
- Chair of Professional Executive Committee (PEC)
- Secretary of Local Medical Committee
- Director or Associate Director of Postgraduate Education
- Strategic Health Authority Director/Chief Executive
- Clinical Director
- Clinical Governance Lead
- RCGP Faculty Chair
- Head of Department of Primary Care (Health Education Institution)
- Director of Services (Community Trust)

Any clinician, before appointment to a managerial role, must demonstrate the managerial competence to undertake what is required in that role: training and support should be made available by trusts and PCTs.

Challenges for clinical managers

A number of challenges present themselves to practitioners who find themselves in a management role, predominantly problems relating to that familiar trio of knowledge, skills, and attitudes. But of equal importance is the thorny prerequisite of protected time. Most of the management roles listed in Box 1.1 are part-time posts with responsibilities discharged over a few sessions per week. The fragmentary nature of this commitment is necessary if practitioners are both to remain in practice and to manage – the central tenet of this book. A problem arises, though, when management becomes subservient to the demands and pressures of clinical practice. Nipping out to a meeting between surgeries, home visits, and prescriptions is unacceptable and does not lead to considered, rational, and effective decision making. Lamentably, this bolt-on approach to management responsibility is endemic in the NHS, particularly amongst doctors, exhausting the individuals concerned and frustrating our professional management colleagues.

It may be that the failure to protect time sufficiently stems from a distrust and undervaluing of management and managers. The preoccupation of managers with systems, resource allocation, and accountability is anathema to professionally autonomous practitioners focused on the best interests of the patient in front of them. The reverse is also true, of course, and the persistent and recurrent failure of doctors and others to engage with management and managers is rooted in this clash of value systems. For a clinician to transfer to 'the dark side' is an act of bravery and risks alienation or ridicule from colleagues. Such suspicion is underpinned by a fundamental misconception of the organisational structures in which we work, where managing 'alongside' in a coaching or collaborative role is frequently a more successful strategy than the top–down approach of traditional hierarchical management.

Doctors and other practitioners can be forgiven their ignorance of the structure and processes of the systems in which they work as, despite repeated calls for change by organisations such as the British Association of Medical Managers, the theory and skills of management have not historically been taught to any great degree at either postgraduate or undergraduate level. Not only that, training and development on the job – the most useful place to learn – has been notable by its absence. There are, though, signs of change.

Fortunately, the NHS has woken up to the needs of its employees, and the Modernisation Agency, the leading edge of the organisation, now provides a number of opportunities in management and leadership. The Agency currently bases its developmental work around three strands: 'improving services', 'building organisations', and 'developing people'.

'Developing people' sets out a raft of provisions aiding the growth of clinical leadership roles, chief executives, PEC members, Board chairs, and practice managers. The, perhaps unfortunately entitled, 'three at the top' programme was designed to improve working relationships between PCT management teams. In addition, there is a National and Regional PCT development programme and a Leadership Centre for Health, devised to aid succession planning in the NHS, which went live in October 2003. There are other professional training opportunities too, of which the RCGP's own leadership programme is an excellent example.

In postgraduate education, General Practice in particular continues to struggle to define a curriculum, but management is increasingly recognised as an important component[8] and attempts have been made to define the management competencies necessary for Primary Care.[9] However, at the level of the undergraduate, likewise in nursing, activity in this area is limited.[10]

Management and leadership

So what is management? *Getting things done through influencing others*[11] is a good holistic starting point, although reductionists would want to break this definition down into its component task-orientated parts (see Box 1.2).

In management jargon, carrying out the tasks in Box 1.2 can be termed

---

Box 1.2 **The tasks of management.**
- Planning
- Allocating resources
- Co-ordinating the work of others
- Motivating staff
- Monitoring output
- Taking responsibility for the process

transactional leadership; that is, managing the complexities of today without necessarily concerning oneself with future developments outside the confines of the immediate operating environment. In the final chapter of this book, we explore leadership in more detail and will be concentrating on *transformational* leadership; that is, recognising the need for revitalisation, creating a new vision, and institutionalising change. Or in other words, shaping tomorrow.

Good management will inevitably involve some form of leadership and there are as many different definitions of leadership as there are leaders. Kenneth Calman offered this one in his farewell speech on stepping down as Chief Medical Officer:[12]

> *Leadership requires knowing where you want to go, taking people with you, and giving sufficient time and energy to make it happen.*

There are, of course, many different leadership styles and success may depend on knowing which one to use in each circumstance.[13] Attempts have been made to define the core competencies necessary for a clinical leader and a typical framework appeared in the *BMJ* careers supplement recently[14] (see Box 1.3). Note the need for credibility – what Weber[15] might have called *legitimacy* – and specialist knowledge; attributes that are only readily accessible to the health care professional being managed.

Box 1.3 **Core competencies of a clinical leader.**
- Credibility
- Insight
- Strategic vision
- Influencing, networking, and building support for change
- Developing and implementing systems, policies, and plans for change
- Developing individual performance and potential
- Developing team and corporate working
- Personal qualities and integrity
- Specialist knowledge

Why should Primary Care practitioners involve themselves with management?

So health care is complex, change in the NHS is occurring at an unprecedented pace, and resource decisions are being made nearer to the patient than ever before. The Griffiths Report[16] underlined, as far back as 1983, that 'the nearer the management process gets to the patient, the more important it becomes for doctors to be looked upon as natural managers'. Twenty years on, it feels normal to apply the same dictum to nurses and the allied health care professions. Indeed, it would be difficult to envisage a situation where doctors and nurses were not central to management within the health service.

So what exactly do Primary Care practitioners bring to management situations?

Firstly, there are core transferable skills. The analytical skills of diagnosis, communication skills honed by years of dealing with patients from all walks of life, and the experience of working within multiprofessional teams all reap immediate rewards when applied to the management situation. Drucker[17] identified five characteristics of the effective executive that also transfer across well from our clinical working lives:

1. Time management.
2. Identifying what we want to contribute to an organisation.
3. Identifying where and how to apply an individual's strengths to best effect.
4. Setting the right priorities.
5. Effective decision making.

Secondly, if resources are to be applied appropriately to best advantage, insider knowledge is essential. That is, if decision making is to be effective, those decisions must be informed and who is better informed than the individuals working with the results of those decisions, the professionals themselves?

> David is an Associate Director in a busy department of Postgraduate General Practice. Following an inspiring meeting he attended recently at the Royal College of General Practitioners (RCGP), he decided that it would be a good idea if all training practices participated in the College's Quality Practice Award. Full of good intentions and determined to improve the quality of health care and training in his area, he announced this at the annual trainers conference. The result: uproar, a torrent of outraged emails, and calls for his resignation. David is puzzled by the response. Isn't what he is proposing for the good of everyone?

Third is the need to manage within the particular and peculiar structure of our professional organisations. Henry Minztberg[18] identified four basic organisational structures:

1. The entrepreneurial start up.
2. The machine bureaucracy.
3. The professional organisation.
4. The *ad hocracy*.

Doctors, and to a lesser extent nurses, tend to work in *professional organisations*, the generic structure of which is illustrated in Figure 1.1. The key feature of such an organisation is that the large operating core, comprising the professionals themselves, is skilled, self-developing, and self-reliant. There is little autocracy and management is focused on support and co-ordination rather than on dictating the needs of the organisation from what Mintzberg terms the *strategic apex*. Who better to manage 'alongside' than a fellow professional? To act otherwise runs the risk of creating destructive tension, as the professional will resist any attempt to define or rationalise his or her skills (by the techno-structure) or dictate what he or she is to do (from the strategic apex) because this erodes professional autonomy. Just look at what happened to David and his Postgraduate Department in our second example. Change in the professional organisation results from a cumulative wisdom seeping in over a number of years as new members join with slightly differing sets of values from their predecessors. Change is a slow process built on what professionals internalise and take with them from their professional training rather than something that is dictated from above. More on Mintzberg and organisational structures in Chapter 11.

Figure 1.1 **The professional organisation**

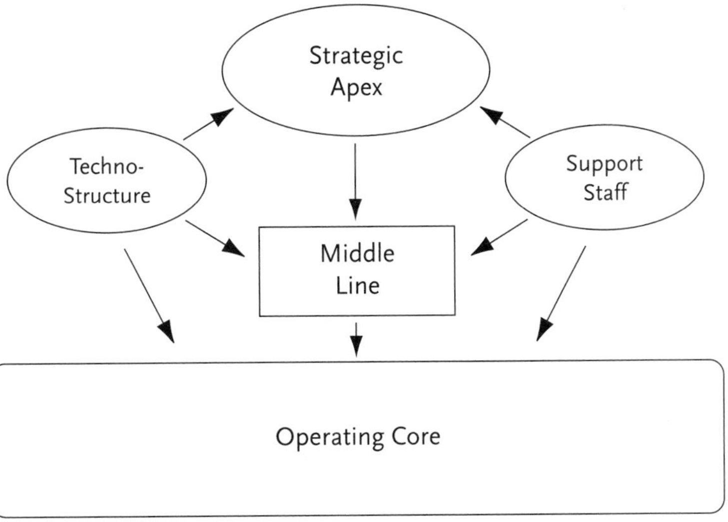

From Henry Mintzberg *Structure in Fives: designing effective organisations.*

Finally, there is the need to manage change effectively by managing the *context* – that is, the sources of influence, the history, and the key players – the *content* – what change is being brought about – and the *process*. Again, the best placed people to manage this activity are those very professionals involved in delivering the changes, a point that was further illuminated by Pettigrew et al[19] in their study of the achievement of strategic service change by health care organisations in the UK. Eight interlinked factors served to delineate top from bottom and the key factors for success appeared to be:

- quality and coherence of local policy
- key people leading change (especially a multidisciplinary team)
- co-operative interorganisational networks
- supportive organisational structure, including the managerial subculture
- environmental pressure that was moderate, predictable, and long-term
- simplicity and clarity of goals and priorities
- positive pattern of managerial and clinical relations
- fitting between the change agenda and the locale.

As will be apparent, all of the above can be enhanced by involving 'coal face' practitioners in the management process, with perhaps the exception of the 'predictable environmental pressure'. Whether the latter can be influenced is debatable, although it might conceivably be achieved through increasing professional representation in government, or for governments to resist the temptation to manage professional organisations as machine bureaucracies.

Conclusion

Management is an activity, not a profession. This practical handbook acknowledges that fact and serves to emphasise that there is a manager in all of us provided we are kitted up with the skills to perform the job. Health care provision and the professional organisations associated with its delivery require good management, and good management requires the committed involvement of health care professionals. Clinicians have the transferable skills and inside knowledge, work within organisations that demand their involvement in management, and are best placed to bring about change, itself an NHS 'specialty'. The argument for health care professionals as managers is compelling. And if you remain unconvinced, ask yourself: What would be the consequences of *not* being involved?

Try this at home

What did you achieve this week through influencing others?

- How did you do it?
- How might you have done it better?

Observe someone in a management position that you respect.

- What skills do you see them employ?
- How might you set about acquiring those skills?

References

1. Plesk P, Greenhalgh T. The challenge of complexity in health care. *BMJ* 2001; **323**: 625–628.
2. Edwards N, Marshall M, McLellan A, Abbasi K. Doctors and managers: a problem without a solution? *BMJ* 2003; **326**: 609–610.
3. Berwick D. A primer on the improvement of systems. *BMJ* 1996; **312**: 619–622.
4. Milburn A. Devolution Day for the NHS. [Press release 2002/0167.] Department of Health, 2002.
5. General Practitioners Committee/Royal College of General Practitioners. *Good Medical Practice for General Practitioners*. London: RCGP, 2002.
6. Laming L. *Inquiry into the death of Victoria Climbié*. London: Stationery Office, 2003.
7. Kennedy I. Public Inquiry into Children's Heart Surgery at the Bristol Royal Infirmary 1984–1995. In: *Learning from Bristol*. London: Stationery Office, 2001.
8. Swanwick T, Chana N. *The Study Guide for General Practice Training*. Abingdon: Radcliffe Medical Press, 2003.
9. Desombre T, Macfarlane F. Doctors in management: an approach to developing competence. *Education for Primary Care* 2002; **13(4)**: 433–444.
10. McClelland S, Jones K. Management education for undergraduate doctors. A survey of medical schools. *Journal of Management in Medicine* 1997; **11(5-6)**: 335–341.
11. Simpson J. Doctors and management – why bother? *BMJ* 1994; **309**: 1505–1508.
12. Calman K. Lessons from Whitehall. *BMJ* 1998; **317**: 1718–1720.
13. Goleman D. Leadership that gets results. *Harvard Business Review* 2000; **Mar–Apr**: 78–90.
14. Empey D, Peskett S, Lees P. Medical leadership. *BMJ Careers* 2002; **325**: s191.
15. Weber M. The Types of Legitimate Domination. In: Wittich C (ed). *Economy and Society*. Berkeley: University of California Press, 1998.
16. Griffiths. *NHS Management Inquiry*. London: DHSS, 1983.
17. Drucker P. *The Effective Executive (Revised)*. New York: Harper Business, 2002.
18. Mintzberg H. *Structure in Fives: designing effective organisations*. Harlow: Prentice Hall, 1992.
19. Pettigrew A, Ferlie E, McKee L. *Shaping Strategic Change: making change in large organisations: the case of the National Health Service*. London: Sage, 1992.

Further reading

Blanchard K, Zigarmi P, Zigarmi D. *Leadership and the One Minute Manager*. Glasgow: William Collins, 1987.

Riley J. *Helping Doctors Who Manage: learning from experience*. London: Kings Fund, 1998.

Modernisation Agency website: www.modernnhs.nhs.uk.

Chapter 2

Making the Right Choice:
Effective and Legal Recruitment and Selection

Antony Americano

 KEY MESSAGES

- Equal opportunities compliance is a key element of recruitment and selection supported by a significant body of legislation.
- The job description, person specification, and application form are the core documents of the recruitment process. A good person specification is essential to effective selection.
- A range of advertising options exist. Advertisements must be clear, honest, and legal.
- Shortlisting based on the person specification helps limit the number of candidates interviewed.
- Interviewing is one of the most popular forms of selection and can be effective when structured.
- A range of other selection instruments exist, but these should be used with care and only by trained individuals.

Introduction

It is people that make the difference to organisations, and in General Practice, to the quality of patient care. The selection of staff is one of the most important tasks a health professional will carry out, but it is the one that is most often rushed, fitted in around a list of competing demands. This is a false economy, as dealing with the consequences of poor selection can be infinitely more time consuming. This chapter tackles the fundamentals of good recruitment practice and, by providing a clear structure to follow, will assist you in developing the skills needed to make the 'right choice'. Following a structured process will not only greatly enhance your chance of making a successful selection, it should help avoid, or defend against, legal challenge. The process is also transferable to other types of selection, for example those concerned with promotion or transfer opportunities.

The principles of equal opportunities underpin effective recruitment and selection and so it is here that we begin. These principles will assist us in drawing up the core documentation of recruitment and selection, namely the *job description* and *person* (sometimes called *employee*) *specification*. Next, we will need to advertise to attract appropriate candidates and lastly, we will explore the key issues in the selection of staff.

Understanding equal opportunities

What do we mean when we talk about equal opportunities in recruitment? Equal opportunity principles are about treating everyone fairly. They are also about recognising that everyone is different and respecting the value that this difference brings. Patients come from a diversity of backgrounds and reflecting this in your workforce will improve communication and understanding. Equal opportunity principles ensure that everyone has an equal **chance**, which means sometimes treating people differently. We will explore this issue further in discussing the different stages of recruitment and selection.

Why are equal opportunities in recruitment and selection important? There are a number of reasons and together they form a compelling argument for incorporating equal opportunities practices into recruitment and selection:

- **Legal requirements**. The law regulates how we behave when recruiting in respect of sex, marital status, gender reassignment, race, nationality, ex-offenders, religion, sexual orientation and disability. At the time of writing, legislation outlawing discrimination on the grounds of age is being drafted.
- **Competitive markets**. We must not forget that as a manager we want to get the best person for the job. Allowing irrelevant factors to cloud this judgement may seriously affect your ability to recruit successfully in the competition for talent.
- **Social reasons**. For many, the strong argument for equal opportunities lies simply in the fact that it is a moral duty to treat everyone fairly and show respect for all.
- **Added value**. If your workforce reflects your local community, this is likely to enhance your credibility as a health care provider. Your workforce is also likely to have skills and knowledge that will improve service provision; e.g. language skills, experience of disability.

Getting to grips with the core recruitment documentation

Well drafted documentation is an important way of improving decision making. Recent research demonstrates that job descriptions are widely used by over 80% of employers. This figure is higher in the public sector. The prevalence of person specifications is just under 75% and again this figure rises when looking only at the public sector.[1]

Job description

The job description is quite simply a list of the duties to be undertaken in a particular role. The development of a job description is a useful first step to a range of other tasks, such as producing a person specification and writing an advert. Where do you start? There are various approaches and which one you choose depends largely on whether there is a current job holder.

Assuming you are writing a job description for an existing role, you can use several methods. Whichever you use, ensure the job holder understands the process in order to avoid unnecessary anxiety.

- The simplest method is to ask the job holder to draft a list of duties and then to sit with them and refine this into a job description.
- If the job holder is new or unsure, ask them to keep a diary of activities for a couple of weeks.
- Alternatively, you could observe and note down the activities in a particular day or week. The length of time will depend on the complexity of the job.

You will also have to consider those tasks that happen less frequently but are nevertheless important; e.g. annual budget setting, annual returns to the Primary Care Trust or Department of Health. This list can be produced from memory, group discussion, or by scrutinising files.

If the post is new, consider the following process:

- Think about scenarios and situations in which the job holder will have to take responsibility and analyse the tasks that are required.
- Consider to whom the job holder should report and for whom, or for what, they are responsible.
- With whom does the job holder interact internally and externally?
- As above, consider tasks that arise infrequently but are still important.

The job description cannot cover every aspect of a job and it is usual practice to add a clause stating:

> This job description can only detail the main areas of work and you will be expected to carry out other tasks broadly similar to those above.

Of course, to keep yourself within the law, you must use this clause reasonably. Were you to add a large number of different duties or require very different skills or much higher responsibilities, you should consult on these changes with the member of staff and seek agreement. To confirm your right to seek such changes to the job description, another clause is often added:

> The (Practice, Organisation) reserves the right to change this job description in the light of the changing needs of the work and/or advances in technology.

Again, this clause should be used reasonably and it is always advisable to consult staff before changing a job description. They may have genuine objections or better alternatives! For a standard job description template see Figure 2.1.

Figure 2.1 **Standard template for a job description**

JOB DESCRIPTION
Job title:
Grade:
Reporting to:
Responsible for:
Summary of duties
Main duties
1. —
2. —
3. —
This job description can only detail the main areas of work and you will be expected to carry out other tasks broadly similar to the above.
The (Practice, Organisation) reserves the right to change this job description in the light of the changing needs of the work and/or advances in technology.

Person specification

A well-drafted person specification is the key to effective and legal recruitment. It contains essential job-related criteria that do not unlawfully discriminate and will differentiate between those who will and will not perform well in the role. The drafting of selection criteria prior to exposure to candidates is helpful in demonstrating an objective approach.

The objection to this formalisation of selection often centres on the exclusion of intuition or 'gut feeling'. At their best, intuition and 'gut feeling' tap subconsciously into a wealth of experience of both good and bad perform-ance.[2] The person specification assists you to draw consciously on this experi-ence and verbalise your opinions. At their worst, intuition and 'gut feeling' are founded on prejudice and cognitive shortcuts that are prone to distortion.[3] Remember, if your processes are challenged legally it is no defence to reply along the lines of 'I have done this job for 20 years and I know when someone is good'.

> Dr Anya, a black post-doctoral research assistant, and Dr Lawrence, the same but white, were based at the University of Oxford. They were both short-listed for a new post-doctoral research post at the University from a pool of 26 applicants. The three-person interview panel included Dr Anya's post-doctoral supervisor, Dr Roberts. Dr Roberts had already formed an adverse view of Dr Anya's suitability for the position and communicated this to a senior panel member. Dr Lawrence was appointed to the post and Dr Anya complained to an employment tribunal of unlawful direct race discrimination.
>
> The case was fought up to the Court of Appeal, a senior court. The senior court took the view that Dr Anya had been treated less favourably. It remitted the case for a rehearing. The Court was influenced by the breach of the University's own policies: no person specification was drawn up until minutes before the interview and no references had been taken up on the candidates. The Court emphasised that breaches of an organisation's own policy, especially concerning person specifications, were a serious matter and likely to lead to inferences of discrimination.
>
> Anya vs University of Oxford and another (2001)

Essential and desirable. The criteria on a person specification are often divided into *essential* and *desirable* items. It is best to minimise desirable criteria, as these may introduce an element of subjectivity and can therefore expose you to claims of discrimination. If a criterion is not essential for the job, desirable items may be seen as raising artificial barriers causing indirect discrimination. On a practical level, over-qualified candidates may become bored and demotivated.

Weighting. It is possible to weight a criterion so that it has a greater influence on the selection decision. One way of doing this is to make it mandatory that the successful candidate fully meets a particular criterion. Alternatively, if responses to questions are being scored, a criterion may be allocated higher marks. If weighting is to be used, the method should be agreed from the outset, before applications are received, and not during the process. This will protect you against allegations that you introduced the weighting rule to exclude certain people.

During recruitment. The person specification is particularly valuable during recruitment. Providing information on the key skills, knowledge, and experience that you are looking for in the advertisement will allow applicants to decide whether they can meet these criteria and therefore whether to apply. While never completely effective, this information should reduce the number of unsatisfactory applications. At interview, clear selection criteria will keep you focused on the requirements of the job. Otherwise it is possible to be swayed by more extrovert or attractive candidates at the expense of those who are quieter but more competent. This phenomenon is called the *halo* effect, where one desirable trait positively influences the evaluation of others. The converse is the *horns* effect, where negative influence occurs.

How do you write a person specification? Not surprisingly, the starting point is the job description. To decide the competencies to perform a job, we need to know what the job holder will do. We can then analyse these tasks to decide the selection criteria for the job. One method is *significant incident analysis*; think of important situations the job holder will have to handle and consider what skills, knowledge, experience, and so on would be needed to do this well. Figure 2.2 provides a standard template for recording selection criteria. The guidance that follows will help you in selecting those criteria.

Figure 2.2 **Standard template for a person specification**

PERSON SPECIFICATION		
Job title:		
Criteria	Essential	Desirable
Skills, Abilities, Knowledge		
Experience		
Qualifications		
Personal qualities		

Skills. A skill is something you can be trained in, though you may have a natural proficiency for a certain area. Common skills required at work include numeracy, communication, and computer literacy. However, for selection criteria to be truly effective, we need to be much more specific. Take numeracy for example; is this required in order to add stationery orders, manage a budget, or to undertake statistical research? Communication, too, is a wide skill area. What particular area is relevant for the job in question? Is it negotiation, counselling, or sensitively handling upset or difficult patients? When it comes to IT skills, are we looking for a proficient user or a systems administrator?

Abilities. These are similar to skills but are often used when the skill itself may not be present. Instead, evidence is sought that the individual has sufficient transferable skills to be able to undertake the role and develop. For example, when filling a first-line management role you may be considering staff who have not directly managed before. Your criterion may then be, 'The ability to manage staff'. An individual may give you examples of courses they have attended, books they have read, and lessons they have learnt from others. They may also be able to draw on experience of assisting temporary staff or colleagues, sitting on selection panels, and taking a lead on a project.

Knowledge. This usually refers to learning of facts and figures, either through study or experience; e.g. knowledge of National Health Service (NHS) financial regulations, knowledge of diabetes management. Sometimes a 'working knowledge' is requested to indicate that evidence of the application of the knowledge is required.

Experience. This is an important criterion but one that can be misused through the application of an arbitrary requirement for the number of years served. Can you justify the requirement for ten years' experience? What is it that is learnt in the second five years that cannot be acquired in the first? Unjustifiable requirements for number of years experience can constitute unfair discrimination and may cut out talented individuals with quality experience. Instead, stick to *minimum years* requirements and specify the type of experience you would have expected to be gained; e.g. 'Two years' experience of practice management to have included budget and premises management and the management of reception and administration services'.

Qualifications. For some roles, qualifications may be considered essential; e.g. Registered Nurse, ENB practice qualification. However, general qualifications gained after leaving school may have little bearing on someone's skills 20 years later. Criteria such as O Level/GCSE Maths and English are often used, unwisely, as shortcuts to skills such as numeracy and literacy. But the reality of an applicant's level of skill can be disappointing, whilst experience gained at work may be more relevant and indicative of their ability. Additionally, you must consider the equivalence of qualifications obtained in other countries. This is not an easy task for small organisations and it may be necessary to ask the candidate to provide evidence of equivalence.

Personal qualities. Personal attributes can make the difference between an effective and ineffective employee. This is the oil that helps the other elements work. Typical criteria are initiative, team skills, and a commitment to professional development.

Try this at home

Write your own job description, or that of a close colleague. Now produce a person specification using the format and advice above. Having put it down for a while, read the document through. Is it clear? Can you think of unambiguous questions you can ask to test each criterion? If you cannot think of a question to test a particular criterion, this is a good indicator that you need to draft that criterion again.

Pass the person specification and job description to a colleague to read. Do they agree with you? Even if they agree, do they understand the same thing as you do about each criterion? When interviewing with each other it is always wise to reach a shared understanding of what you are looking for prior to shortlisting and interviewing.

Curriculum Vitae or application forms?

You will need to make a choice about how you receive information from candidates. Curriculum Vitaes (CVs) require less administration from an employer's point of view and are less work for a candidate. Application forms, supported by job descriptions and person specifications, allow you to request more job-relevant information and can speed up shortlisting. They can also cover legal best practice issues by requesting information for equal opportunities monitoring purposes, advising candidates of the consequences of providing false information, and agreeing to the processing of their data under the Data Protection Act 1998. They do require more administration by employers and greater input from candidates. Their inclusion will also add time to the selection process.

Advertising

When recruiting, you need to attract a sufficient number of suitable applicants in order to make a choice. Remember that recruitment is a two-way process. A good applicant can apply for many jobs. Why should they apply to you? By providing information about you as an employer, the duties and requirements of the job, and the benefits, you initiate a selling process that should also continue during the interview. This information can form part of an advertisement that can be placed in a wide range of places, depending on the job and the job market.

Word of mouth recruitment alone is open to challenge as being discriminatory. If your workforce is not representative of the community you serve, word of mouth recruitment is more likely to replicate the existing situation. It is also unlikely to provide you with a good range of candidates.

Local advertising in shops, job centres may be particularly useful for part-time and non-professional posts.

Local and national media and professional press. Budget is an issue here, as advertisements in national and professional media can cost thousands of pounds for a reasonably sized box. Of course, the cost is justified if this is the only way to attract the right candidates. Rates are usually based on a single column centimetre, so be economical with your words!

Internet-based advertising. There is an increasing use of job boards – websites specialising in recruitment. Examples of these include: www.jobsgopublic.co.uk, www.jobsin.co.uk/jobsin/health, and www.monster.co.uk, as well as web-based journals, such as www.bmjcareers.com. If you are considering this method, visit the sites and look around. Are there similar employers or jobs? What information do these employers provide? If you have your own website, it is often helpful to link to this from the job board to allow candidates to learn more about you.

When drafting an advertisement be clear, honest, and legal. In particular, get your point across using as simple language as possible and do not oversell the job or the organisation. The reality soon becomes apparent and a disillusioned employee is of no value. Do not use language that could be deemed to be discriminatory; e.g. calling a vacancy by a gender-specific title, such as 'handyman', 'cleaning lady', etc.

What to put in an advert
- Tasks/duties of the job
- Key skills and experience sought
- Something unique or interesting about the practice/organisation
- Job location
- Reward package (salary, allowances, annual leave, pension)
- Job tenure (e.g. contract length)
- Application procedure

This information will minimise the chances of a candidate rejecting a job offer later on in the process due to a mismatch in expectations that could have been identified earlier.

Selection

Shortlisting

Having advertised, you may receive more candidates than you would want to interview. Even if this were not the case, you would not want to waste time by interviewing individuals who were obviously unsuitable. To avoid this situation, shortlisting is carried out. A decision is made about the number of candidates you want to interview. Candidates' CVs or application forms are compared against the person specification and a written note of how well they meet it is made. Those most closely meeting the person specification criteria are accepted for interview. If requested, it is good practice to give feedback to unsuccessful applicants.

Selection interview

By far the most widely used method of selection is the interview.[4] While early research cast doubt on the predictive validity of the selection interview – i.e. whether it would select a competent candidate – more recent work has confirmed that the interview, where structured, does offer good predictive validity.[5] It is good practice to ensure that interviewers have had training in selection, but any training you commission should be carried out by appropriately skilled personnel and cover the legal aspects of recruitment and selection.

Structured interviewing builds on the discussion earlier in the chapter on job descriptions and person specification. Use the person specification to produce questions to explore the candidate's ability to fulfil the criteria. Ask all candidates the same questions. Some small wording change is acceptable to recognise, for example, that a candidate does not have direct experience in a particular area but may have transferable skills. Follow-up questions should also be asked to probe the quality of the response (see Figure 2.3). Follow-up questions may differ between candidates so long as they continue to probe the same person specification criterion. Do not make assumptions about one candidate that are not made about another, unless you have an objective and discrimination-free reason. For example, questioning a woman about her ability to work early evenings should not assume she bears childcare responsibilities.

Behavioural interviewing is one approach that looks at past experience as an indicator of likely future performance. Its purpose is to seek examples where similar skills, knowledge, or aptitudes have been demonstrated in other roles and to identify how well these were handled.

Figure 2.3 **Funnelling questions technique**

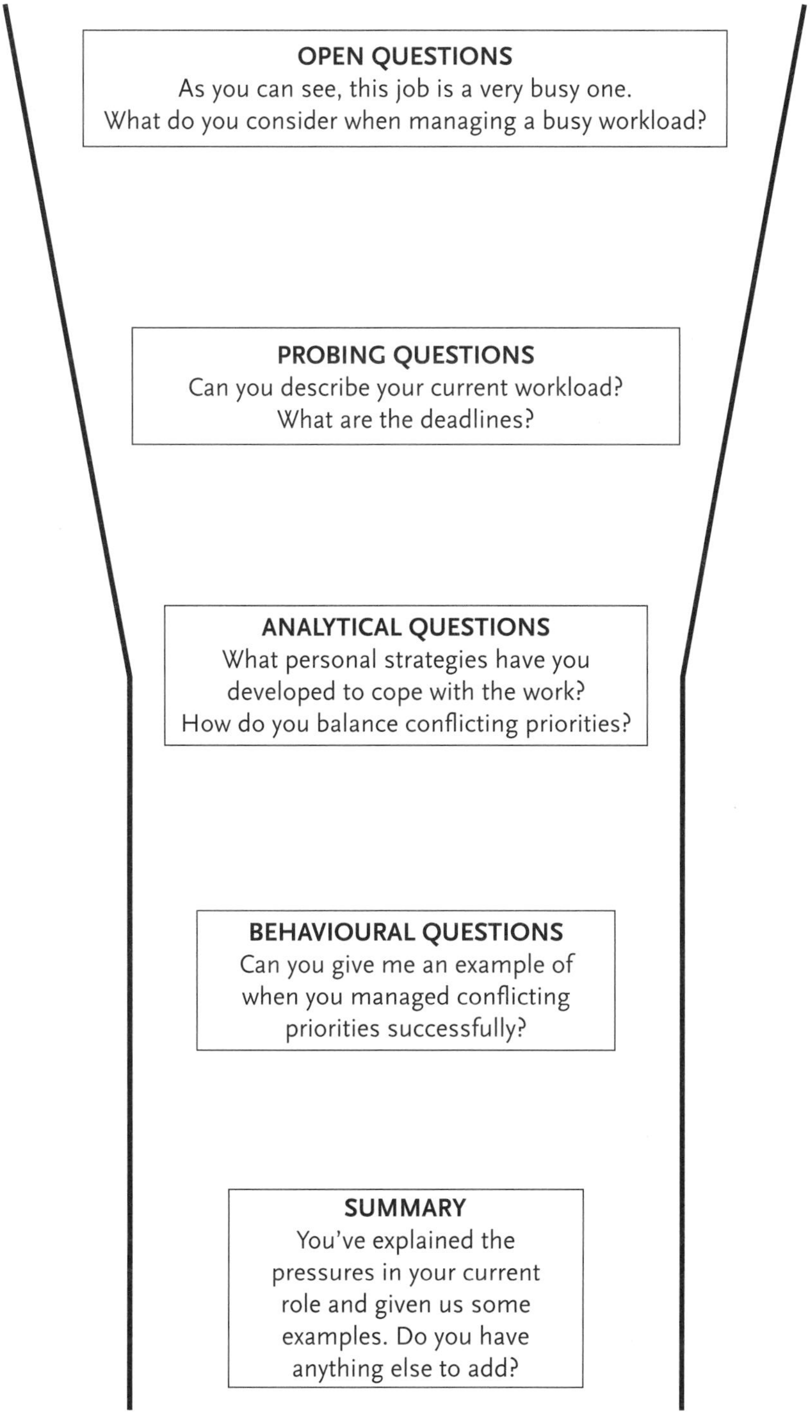

OPEN QUESTIONS
As you can see, this job is a very busy one.
What do you consider when managing a busy workload?

PROBING QUESTIONS
Can you describe your current workload?
What are the deadlines?

ANALYTICAL QUESTIONS
What personal strategies have you
developed to cope with the work?
How do you balance conflicting priorities?

BEHAVIOURAL QUESTIONS
Can you give me an example of
when you managed conflicting
priorities successfully?

SUMMARY
You've explained the
pressures in your current
role and given us some
examples. Do you have
anything else to add?

References

There are two approaches to references. The first is to use them as part of the interview process in order to explore candidates' strengths and weaknesses. This approach is only really fair if you do this for all candidates and, in practice, it can be difficult to obtain references for all candidates in time for the interview. You must also make it clear to the referees that information that they provide will be disclosed to candidates otherwise you will fall foul of the Data Protection Act 1998.

The other approach is to take up references after the selection and to use these as a confirmation of factual information provided and to pick up any warning signs on performance and attendance. The area of references is now more legally complex than ever before and a full exploration of this subject is outside the remit of this chapter. There is more advice available on the Advisory, Conciliation and Arbitration Service (ACAS) website (www.acas.gov.uk).

Whichever approach you take to references, a structured reference, that is a form asking specific questions based on the person specification and key areas of conduct and attendance, is recommended.

Disability

> Mr Keane was interviewed for a job as a part-time medical records clerk for Lincolnshire NHS Hospitals Trust. Mr Keane is deaf. He did not succeed in his application for the post because he could not answer incoming telephone calls. He complained to an Employment Tribunal of disability discrimination.
>
> Was this decision lawful? What action, if any, should have been considered before taking such a decision?
>
> The tribunal (Keane vs. Lincolnshire NHS Hospitals Trust (ET, 2002)) decided that the employer should have made reasonable adjustments concerning the use of the telephone that would have overcome or reduced his difficulties. Despite Mr Keane having made several suggestions, no action had been taken. The tribunal found that Mr Keane had been discriminated against on the grounds of his disability.

In relation to disability, the law requires that you make *reasonable adjustments* to facilitate a disabled person when attending an interview and in their employment. What is reasonable will depend on the size of your organisation and the resources available to you. The best way of finding out what adjustments a disabled person may require is to ask them, as they tend to be the expert on themselves. Questioning around the issue of disability needs to be considered carefully. Avoid asking personal questions about a person's disability, such as, 'Were you born like that?' You could ask, 'Does your disability affect your ability to do this job?' Visit the Disability Rights Commission website for further guidance (www.drc-gb.org).

Other selection instruments

If selection tests are used, they should be specifically related to job requirements and should measure an individual's actual ability to do the work. A scoring system should be agreed before the test is delivered and the weighting that the test will carry, in relation to other selection methods, clarified.

Psychometric testing is often used by larger organisations and can focus on either ability (numerical, spatial awareness, critical reasoning) or personality tests. These tests need to be delivered and interpreted by qualified individuals.

Work sample tests are tests that ask an individual to carry out, under assessment, a sample of a task on the job description. A typing test is the most well-known and used example.

Assessment centres bring together a range of these and other techniques. They do, however, require considerable time and money to set up, as well as professional input.

A number of websites (addresses below) will provide you with more information on selection tools.

References

1. IRS Employment Review. Setting the Tone: job descriptions and person specifications. 2003; 42–48.
2. Bower B. Seeing through experts eyes: ace decision makers may perceive distinctive worlds (intuition and experience in decision making). *Science News* 1998; **154(3)**: 44-46.
3. Tversky A, Kahneman D. Judgement under uncertainty: Heuristics and biases. *Science* 1974; **185**: 1124–1131.
4. Dipboye S. Structured Selection Interview – Why do they work? Why are they under-utilised? In: *The International Handbook of Selection and Assessment*. Anderson N, Herriott P (eds). New York: John Wiley & Sons Ltd, 1997.
5. Schmidt FL, Hunter JE. The validity of and utility of selection methods in personnel psychology. Practical and theoretical implications of 85 years of research findings. *Psychological Bulletin* 1998; **124(2)**: 262–274.

Further reading

Most people have access to the web nowadays and there is a wealth of content available on equalities in general and recruitment specifically.

Commission for Racial Equality The Commission for Racial Equality is a publicly funded nongovernmental body set up under the Race Relations Act 1976 to tackle racial discrimination and promote racial equality: www.cre.gov.uk.

Disability Rights Commission The Disability Rights Commission (DRC) is an independent body, established by Act of Parliament to eliminate discrimination against disabled people and promote equality of opportunity: www.drc-gb.org.

Equal Opportunities Commission The Equal Opportunities Commission is the leading agency working to eliminate sex discrimination in 21st Century Britain: www.eoc.org.uk.

CIPD The website of the Chartered Institute of Personnel & Development: www.cipd.co.uk.

ACAS The Advisory, Conciliation and Arbitration Service – a government-sponsored body that provides a wide range of advice on employee relations: www.acas.gov.uk.

Department of Trade & Industry (DTI) The government department responsible for employment legislation. It provides a wealth of guidance notes on many issues including recruitment: www.dti.gov.uk/er/index.htm.

A few books, too:

Fullerton J, Kandola R. *Diversity in Action: managing the mosaic (developing strategies)*. London: Royal Paperback, 1998.

Macdougald AN, King P, Jones P, Eveleigh M. *A Tool Kit for Practice Nurses. [Developing Primary Care Series.]* Chichester: Aeneas Press, 2001. *Has a complete set of core competencies for all grades from HCA to I.*

Roberts G. *Recruitment & Selection: a competency approach (developing practice)*. London: Royal Paperback, 1997.

Chapter 3

Appraisal and Performance Management

Julia Whiteman

 KEY MESSAGES

- Appraisal and performance management are different and a clear boundary between the two should be maintained.
- Any appraisal process must be owned by all those involved.
- Appraisal requires well-trained appraisers sympathetically matched to their appraisees.
- There must be agreement to the process of addressing the learning objectives from appraisal with a commitment to life-long learning throughout the organisation.
- Ground rules should be established for the conduct of the appraisal interview, including adequate protected time, a quiet, confidential location, and confidentiality around the content of the discussion.
- Adequate preparation time for the appraisee and the appraiser is essential.

Introduction

This chapter examines the definitions of appraisal and performance management and how they are related in Primary Care. It describes how to set up an appraisal system within a primary health care team and moves on to discuss approaches to your own appraisal and ongoing professional development. Most of the content of the chapter is generic and may be applied to any appraisal taking place within the National Health Service (NHS) at whatever level.

What is appraisal?

Appraisal is a professional process whereby individuals can consider their recent achievements and current challenges in a way that encourages personal development in the context of the work environment. The drive to establish formal appraisal systems in the NHS stemmed from the Department of Health's policy document, *Supporting Doctors, Protecting Patients* that appeared in 1999 (see Further reading).

Appraisal in Primary Care should be thought of as a continuous process whereby a member of the primary health care team reviews and reflects on their work and achievements and discusses this with their appraiser in an appropriately supportive environment. The appraisers themselves need to be trained for their role.

An action or personal learning plan flows from the appraisal discussion and, in General Practice, this should be relevant to the ongoing development of that individual within their primary health care team and the team's work in providing health care to the local community of patients. The critical part then follows. For the appraisal process to have any meaning, the appraisee has to take the action plan forwards, endeavouring to meet the objectives set. The appraisal discussion acts as a catalyst for the appraisee's professional development, building on the quality of care they provide to their patients, enhancing their role in the primary health care team, supporting career development, and contributing to the development of the team as a whole.

What is performance management?

Performance management, by contrast, is the process by which the service provided by an individual is reviewed in the light of a suggestion that it does not reach a standard appropriate to that role or that individual. Unlike the developmental process of appraisal, performance management is very much a structured managerial task conducted according to the performance procedures agreed by the organisation and relevant professional body. It is not a regular cyclical process but one that is used only when necessary to assess and address an individual's performance within their prescribed role.

Why appraisal and performance management must be distinguished

It is important to distinguish clearly between appraisal and performance management – the terms are often used interchangeably – and for that distinction to be clear throughout your organisation. For the appraisal process to work, the context must be one that is developmentally supportive. If the appraisee views the appraisal process as an assessment of their performance then the educational nature of appraisal will be undermined. Even if there is a performance issue relating to the appraisee at the time of their appraisal, they should still be entitled to a developmental appraisal. By the same token, if a performance issue comes to light within the appraisal interview then this cannot be ignored. It will present a sensitive situation, the outcome of which will depend on a number of factors, including the skills of the appraiser, their relationship to the appraisee, the attitude of the appraisee, and the nature of the problem. If needs be, the appraisal should be stopped such that the performance issue can be addressed according to the appropriate procedures. However, it might be possible to continue with the appraisal if the problem can be reviewed, reflected upon, and dealt with in a constructive way through specific objectives in the learning plan and with the appraisee demonstrating a commitment to see it through.

Creating a context for appraisal

At the outset of this chapter we defined appraisal as a mechanism for both individual and organisational development. Individual and organisational development are mutually dependent and a healthy working environment is one with a strong commitment to personal development and life-long learning. An organisation can only move forward and develop if the individuals within it are learning and developing in a constructive way. Senge[1] discusses this in his book, *The Fifth Discipline* highlighting the importance of valuing the people and teams working in an organisation.

With this in mind, an appraisal system should be set in a culture of safety whereby an individual is treated with respect and confidentiality. The method for appraisal must be fair and effective for all team members, comprehensive, and relevant to the appraisees such that they can feel that they own the process and benefit from it. Again, the outcome from the appraisal interviews, namely the contents of the personal learning plans, must be dealt with in a way that demonstrates a commitment to invest in and value all members of the practice team. It is important to remember that appraisal is more than just an interview – it is a cyclical process of reflection, learning, application, and review.

A culture of appraisal and continuing professional development can be developed by:

- including everyone in the team when discussing the objectives of a proposed appraisal system
- involving everyone in setting up the system, including selecting the appraisal model to be followed (see below)
- developing ground rules for the system in consultation with the entire team. Ground rules might include how the appraisal interview will be conducted, how the time will be protected, confidentiality around the appraisal interview, and responsibility for meeting the ongoing developmental needs devised during the appraisal interview by the individuals and the team.

Try this at home

Think about a situation either in your work or your home life, where you are, or have been, part of a group that you find enjoyable, fulfilling, and that achieves its purpose. Try to identify the aspects of this group that help this happen and the role you play contributing to this. What features of this would you want to bring into an appraisal system in your organisation?

Models of appraisal

The two important factors that feed into how the appraisal model is defined are: (i) the relationship of the appraiser to the appraisee; and (ii) how the information discussed in the appraisal interview is collected.

To take the first point, those within a primary health care team available to act as appraisers may or may not be from the same profession/discipline as the appraisee. In addition, they may or may not have line management or indeed employer responsibility for the appraisee. Clearly, the size of the team and therefore the number of people available to act as appraisers will have an impact here, but essentially, the models that can be adopted are:

Peer appraisal. The appraisal is conducted by someone from the same profession or discipline that does not have line management responsibility for the appraisee.

Manager appraisal. The appraiser does have line management responsibility and hence any performance targets set might therefore assume a greater significance.

External appraisal. The appraiser is someone from outside the appraisee's organisation. Whilst such appraisers are likely to be highly experienced, they may well be compromised by a lack of local relevant knowledge about the organisation and the individuals working within it.

Daisy chain appraisal. All members of the team participate in appraising each other across professional and disciplinary boundaries.

With regard to the second point, the information discussed within the appraisal interview can either be selected by the appraisee alone or collected through a previously agreed process. Such a process may include the canvassing of patients or staff for their views on the appraisee's performance. This is known as *360 degree appraisal.* A compromise between the two approaches would be for the appraisee to collect views from colleagues and patients and then select those they wanted to include in their appraisal discussion.

Clearly, 360 degree appraisal allows an opportunity for others to feed into the process, so enriching the information available for discussion at the appraisal interview. 360 degree appraisal needs to be carried out in an agreed and structured manner, preferably with an emphasis on presenting any information in a positive light. The risk with 360 degree appraisal is that feedback may be damaging and hurtful to the appraisee, thus compromising developmental opportunities that might otherwise have presented themselves at the appraisal interview. Ground rules are essential when discussing feedback from colleagues; perhaps that all feedback should be based on direct experience rather than hearsay, that statements should be owned rather than anonymous, and that comments should be positive and constructive, aimed at bringing about improvement, not character assassination!

What skills are necessary as an appraiser?

The success of the appraisal process will largely be dependent upon the skills of those people acting as appraisers. An appraiser needs to be able to listen, to respond sensitively, probing where necessary to aid greater reflection on the part of the appraisee. They should not be judgemental and need to be able to divorce themselves from their own agenda of concerns and challenges, in particular those that might be relevant to the ones being brought to the appraisal discussion by the appraisee.

It is important that the appraiser has sufficient background knowledge to understand the information being presented and discussed by the appraisee. Appraisers need to be trustworthy, to command the respect of those they are appraising, and to be committed to the development of themselves and the team through the appraisal process.

It is recommended that anyone undertaking the role of appraiser should have undergone training for that role that included the opportunity to practise the skills listed above. Such training is readily available through Primary Care Trusts (PCTs) and providers of higher professional education. Anyone trained as an appraiser should have an appreciation of their own personal development, both as a member of the primary health care team and as an appraiser.

Who manages the system and what does this involve?

Regardless of the model selected, someone has to take responsibility to ensure the appraisal system runs smoothly throughout its cycle. Generally, a cycle is taken to last a year with a round of annual appraisals set up at a time convenient to the planning process for practice development. Therefore, it is important that whoever manages this process is aware of the other planning pressures that occur within the year from both the practice's perspective and the PCT's, since the developmental needs identified through appraisal are likely to draw on funding resources that need to be factored into budget planning. Most organisations have an identified period for appraisals that occurs before the start of the run up to the next financial year.

Having identified when the round of appraisals will take place the appraisal manager needs to ensure that there is:

- space available to hold the appraisal interviews
- protected time that is convenient to the appraisees and the appraisers
- sufficient notice given that it is appraisal time again.

Matching the appraiser to the appraisee is a critical part of the process. Clearly, if the model adopted defines who will perform an appraisal then this step is straightforward. However, where this is not the case, there must be an agreed mechanism whereby the appraisee can agree to be appraised by their appointed appraiser and vice versa, whilst ensuring that the workload is appropriately distributed.

Having completed the round of appraisal interviews, the appraisal manager should ensure that the different individual learning plans are collated such that the practice, or organisation, can address the identified learning needs through-out the coming months.

Embarking on your own appraisal

The prospect of an impending appraisal interview can be daunting. Remember, though, the purpose of an appraisal is to help you recognise your ongoing developmental needs within the context of your professional work and life. The appraisal is therefore 100% grounded in reality, both in terms of what is reflected upon and what is decided as an action plan.

If you have already had an appraisal that resulted in a personal learning plan, or have a personal learning plan for another reason, then start by reviewing your progress with that plan. What have you achieved and how has this changed your practice? Why are some things left incomplete? Is this because the objectives were poorly defined, too large to be fully addressed, or has your plan been eclipsed by other events? Such reflection is important, as it will help you create a more focused learning plan in future.

If you are preparing for your first appraisal, you might think that you have not yet put together a personal development or learning plan. This is not the case, even though your plan may not be written in a formal manner. An essential part of the thinking of anyone involved in patient care is to assess and plan for patients' needs and therefore how you, as the primary health care team member, will meet those needs. Your thinking is always underpinned by planning and included in that planning will be how you will set about meeting the needs of your patients at times when you are otherwise unsure.

Try this at home

Think about a recent major event in your domestic life: planning an expensive holiday, moving house, getting married, preparing for the birth of a child. How did you approach this event? What past experience did you draw on? How did you ensure you could cope with the challenges it would present? What did you learn from the experience that you would apply to a similar situation in the future? Try to apply what you have discovered about your planning, experience, and review cycle to how you meet new challenges in your work.

Identifying your personal development and achievements

There are many sources of material that you might use to identify your personal development and achievements. Box 3.1 lists a few that will hopefully help you prepare for your next appraisal.

SWOT analysis – strengths, weaknesses, opportunities, and threats – will give a snapshot profile of where you are currently. It is a useful way of critically appraising your situation as it takes in the positives as well as the negatives and allows you to include your personal as well as your professional life, thereby building up a picture that is personally relevant to you.

PUNS and DENS[2] is a useful tool for discovering educational needs in General Practice. During the working day, doctors or nurses reflect on consultations/transactions with their patients and ask themselves if the patients' needs have been met. If they haven't, then a PUN – the patient's unmet need – has been identified. Later reflection on why you failed to meet their need results in the creation of your DEN – doctor's educational need. The DEN may be knowledge-based – clinical or non-clinical – a skill, or management-based. The DEN can be met by covering the knowledge or skill gap yourself, delegation to another member of the team better equipped to address the problem, or an administrative change to the way you or the practice team function. Whilst PUNS and DENS were originally designed to help doctors develop their clinical practice,

---

Box 3.1 **Possible sources of material to bring to an appraisal.**
- Learning outcomes from previous appraisal/personal learning plan
- SWOT analysis
- PUNS and DENS record
- Significant event analysis record
- 360 degree feedback
- Compliments and complaints
- Outcomes from audits

they are just as useful and relevant to all other members of the team. Frequently, the perception is that our biggest knowledge gap is around clinical facts and detail. In reality it is more often a skill or a practice organisational issue that results in us delivering care that is not to the standard we would like. PUNS and DENS is a useful way of illustrating where developmental needs lie.

Significant events.[3] Anything that has happened that has been out of the ordinary and affected your work either as an individual or as a practice team is a useful educational resource and a good starting point for identifying how and what you might have learnt and how that in turn has influenced your practice. It might be that you have regular practice meetings where things that might have happened differently, successes, and near misses are reviewed as a team. Look back over these meetings and reflect on what you have learnt and how this has changed your practice.

> *A patient has slipped on a wet floor in reception. Although they are not seriously hurt, they are shaken up and their spouse rings to complain later. This is all discussed at the next practice meeting, where the practice manager undertakes to arrange for the lino to be replaced and some non-slip mats to be put down. However, the discussion moves onto the practice's health and safety policy. You know that you have never really looked at the policy, as it has never seemed important. However, now that an incident has occurred you see the importance of it and make a mental note to look it up later.*
>
>   *Reading the policy makes you think that it needs updating to include the changes made to the practice team's roles and responsibilities. Also, some examples would make it seem more real and relevant and therefore a more useful and interesting document.*

360 degree feedback. We are our own sternest critics! We always think of the things we did not do so well, often exaggerating them and allowing them to eclipse our achievements. This is where 360 degree feedback can be very helpful, as others are often quicker to recognise our strengths. Thank you letters, complaints, and other feedback from patients and colleagues are a rich source. Identify your successes and build on them by analysing what went well and how you might use that success in other areas.

Audit now plays an increasingly important part in practice development and professional practice, both clinical and administrative. As with significant incidents, the findings from any audit, and in particular the changes to your practice that have resulted, will be relevant information to bring to your appraisal.

The appraisal interview

The structure and process for the appraisal interview should be agreed in advance. Sufficient time must be available, in a room away from the hustle and bustle of the practice, where both the appraiser and the appraisee feel at ease. While the appraiser's sitting room may seem the simplest and most comfortable option to them, the appraisee might feel that the unfamiliar territory within a domestic context rather than the workplace is inappropriate.

Adequate notice needs to be given to allow time for the appraisee to prepare and collect information to be discussed at the interview. Likewise, the appraiser needs time to assimilate this information before meeting with the appraisee.

A wide range of formats for the appraisal interview is currently in use throughout organisations both within and outside the NHS. Since generally these are the tools for individual and organisational development and are not clinically based, they are widely applicable. An exception here is the GP appraisal forms in use at the time of writing that are very specifically based around the model of *Good Medical Practice.*

The essence of any appraisal form lies in the questions:
- What have you done well?
- ... what have you learnt from this?
- What might you have done differently?
- ... what have you learnt from this?
- What do see as your current challenges or developmental needs?
- How would you like to see your career developing from here?

Whatever framework is selected by the practice it needs to be relevant to the ongoing professional development of the individual professions and disciplines represented within the team. In selecting the framework it is helpful to consider the outcome of the appraisal, namely the personal learning plan. This plan must be of relevance to the individual within the team and to their professional development. Having one appraisal as a team member and another for professional development causes unnecessary duplication and the risk that two different plans could emerge, neither of which capture the development needs of the individual within the context of their contribution to the practice team or their profession.

Any appraisal form adopted should be as simple as possible, to allow for flexibility and to accommodate a range of people using it. Long and complicated forms run the risk that an appraisee may drown, struggling through pages of ever more detailed and thought-stifling questions.

The final point to be made in relation to the appraisal interview is the amount of time needed for the discussion, reflection, and construction of the resulting personal learning plan. How much time is needed? The answer is 'enough'. An appraisal interview cannot be rushed, as this will limit the discussion and reflection that is so essential for making it effective as a developmental exercise. The skill of the appraiser in focusing the discussion, listening actively and probing where necessary will help to keep the appraisal on course. The importance of adequate preparation prior to the interview on behalf of the appraiser and the appraisee cannot be overstated. Having found an appropriate environment for the appraisal in which both the appraiser and the appraisee feel at ease will help to get the process under way swiftly, as will a mutual awareness of the ground rules and boundaries around the appraisal, including confidentiality.

Formulating the action plan from the appraisal interview

The concluding part of the appraisal interview will revolve around formulating an action plan that will underpin the practitioner's development until their next appraisal – usually a period of 12 months. The plan must be one that the appraisee is committed to working on and that they see is going to be of use to them.

In putting together a learning plan it is worthwhile recalling that in order to enhance the chances of achieving set objectives, they should be SMART. That is to say:

- Specific
- Measurable
- Achievable
- Relevant
- Time-bounded.

Let us return to our case study of the practice's health and safety policy. During the appraisal discussion you might discuss how far your thinking had progressed with this project and how you wanted to take it further. Maybe you would know that the PCT had an update in this area arranged for the near future and you were happy to attend the event, feed back, and participate in re-shaping the practice's policy as part of expanding your knowledge and understanding of health and safety.

> *Objectives for the review of the practice's health and safety policy*
> *– To review the practice's health and safety policy with the PCT health and safety lead, discussing how you think it needs improving*
> *– To attend the PCT's update with specific points in mind for clarification*
> *– To access expertise in the PCT for any outstanding points not addressed by the update*

> – To discuss your proposed changes with the practice, to obtain general
> agreement at the meeting scheduled for two weeks after the update
> – To participate in re-writing the policy with the health and safety lead
> and presenting this to the practice team
> – To have the new policy in place within six months

Working towards next appraisal

With the learning plan agreed the appraisal cycle moves into the next stage, where the objectives set are addressed and woven into the practitioner's work as part of the development of services offered by the practice team. It is important to remember that the learning plan cannot possibly cover all the challenges to be faced between agreeing the plan and the next review. All learning, whether it is included in or is in addition to the plan, must be valued, recorded, and acted upon to harness it into the practitioner's growing collection of competencies. Progress on the plan should be reviewed regularly throughout the year and the plan adapted where necessary to take into account unforeseen factors affecting the practitioner, their work, and their learning.

> What did you achieve from health and safety policy work?
> – New policy in place with greater team relevance and ownership
> – Greater personal understanding of the practice's health and safety
> policy
> – Greater understanding of health and safety legislation
> – Experience of working with colleagues to write practice policy – I never
> thought I could do it!
> – Presentation experience at practice meeting – I found I was not as
> nervous as I thought and enjoyed positive feedback afterwards!!
> – Know more people at the PCT and have been invited to participate
> in other events
> . . . and all this from an appraisal!

A final word on appraisal and revalidation for GPs

At the time of writing, the General Medical Council has linked GP appraisal and revalidation by announcing that one route to revalidation would be through five successful annual appraisals using the format laid down for GPs by the Department of Health. How can this be reconciled with all that has been said earlier in this chapter about the developmental nature of appraisal? The answer lies in remembering the underlying principle of appraisal: to encourage the practitioner to reflect upon their work and, in so doing, review and positively adapt their performance. It follows, therefore, that it is the process of the appraisal rather than the content that will support revalidation and the ongoing development of individuals as practitioners, and therefore Primary Care.

References

1. Senge P. *The Fifth Discipline*. New York: Doubleday, 2000.
2. Eve R. *PUNS and DENS: discovering learning needs in general practice*. Oxford: Radcliffe, 2003.
3. Pringle M, Bradley C, Carmichael C, *et al*. *Significant Event Auditing*. [Occasional Paper No. 70.] London: RCGP, 1995.

Further reading

Brookfield S. *Developing Critical Thinkers: challenging adults to explore alternative ways of thinking and acting*. San Francisco: Jossey Bass, 1987.

Department of Health. *Supporting Doctors, Protecting Patients*. London: Department of Health, 1999.

Department of Health. *The NHS Plan*. London: Department of Health, 2000.

General Medical Council. *Revalidation for Doctors: ensuring standards, securing the future*. London: General Medical Council, 2000.

General Practitioners Committee/Royal College of General Practitioners. *Good Medical Practice for General Practitioners*. London: RCGP, 2002.

Pietroni R. *The Toolbox for Portfolio Development*. Oxford: Radcliffe, 2001.

Rughani A. *The GP's Guide to Personal Development Plans*. Oxford: Radcliffe, 2001.

Chapter 4

Effective Team Working

Julia Oxenbury

 KEY MESSAGES

- Teams are groups working together to achieve a common purpose or goal.
- Teams provide a social structure and mutual support.
- Effective teams make better decisions, are more productive, and take more risks.
- Teams form in stages and require a different style of management at each stage.
- Teams contain a mix of roles and require suitable individuals to fill those roles.
- Teams need regular team building to maintain their function.

Introduction

One of the fundamental aspects of Primary Care is that we work in teams. Indeed, the concept of the primary health care team is a common reason offered by GP registrars for having made a career choice of General Practice. It can be a pleasure to work in a team that functions well and immensely rewarding to be involved in a productive and effective unit. However, be warned: there are good teams and bad teams, functional and dysfunctional teams, and, quite frankly, teams from hell.

For a team to be effective, attention should be paid to three sets of needs: those of the *task*, those of the *individuals*, and those of the *team* itself. Co-ordinating these various requirements will achieve harmony and results.

John is a bright enthusiastic new partner, with a Fraser Rose Medal, working in a four-partner rural practice in an idyllic setting. It is just where his wife always wanted to settle down. He has replaced an 'old-school' GP who was happy to offer routine visits to her older patients at their convenience and it was not unusual for her to have three visits after evening surgery. At a practice meeting he tells his partners that his

> *workload needs to be rationalised as he is heading for burnout. There have*
> *already been two informal complaints from elderly patients that he*
> *declined to visit for social reasons. He asks for a practice away day*
> *involving the whole primary health care team to develop a strategy for*
> *visiting...*

Increasingly, we hear stories of problems in practices; more partnerships are dissolving and the traditional units of General Practice are fragmenting. This has been attributed to a number of external factors affecting the functioning of practice teams, namely:

- change in organisational structure; e.g. introduction of Primary Care Organisations
- introduction of Personal Medical Services
- changing work description; e.g. new General Medical Services (GMS) Contract
- changing work patterns; e.g. nurse practitioner role
- increasing job mobility
- increasing numbers of GPs working part-time or with portfolio careers.

Given the context, it has become more important than ever for practitioners to develop not only an insight into what constitutes effective team working but also, how to bring it about. In this chapter we will consider what constitutes a team, the benefits that team working can bring to an organisation, the problems that teams commonly encounter, how teams form, and how they can be built. The chapter will provide the theory behind these headings, offer models of team dynamics, and provide exercises for you to work through. By the end, you should have a greater understanding of how your own team functions.

You may find this chapter particularly helpful if faced with the following circumstances:

- You are about to join a new team.
- You are taking on increased responsibility within your team.
- You are involved in a team building exercise.
- You just want to look at how your team is performing.

What constitutes a team

A team is defined as two or more interacting individuals working together to achieve a common goal or goals. It is important that the group has a stable structure and that the individual members perceive themselves as a team.

Team size

A common question relates to the size of a team. A consensus view from various authors suggests that the optimum size is between 5–12 individuals, with 20 as a maximum for effectiveness. A larger team may comprise a greater array of skills, talents, and available knowledge. However, with increased numbers in a group there is less opportunity for an individual to participate fully and a greater need for effective communication. Larger teams also run the risk of fragmentation and the formation of sub-groups, and research indicates that teams of over 20 appear to have more absenteeism and lower morale.[1]

Common goals

The shared or common goals should only be achievable by the members working together and not as individuals. While individuals may also wish to achieve their own particular objective, it is necessary that all members feel committed to contribute to the attainment of the shared goal.

Social interaction

It is important that the members of a team have some social interaction; that is they have effective communication networks and have some influence over each other. Maslow[2] suggested that people are social animals and have a basic need to interact with others. Teams can provide opportunities for mutual support and fellowship, especially when they succeed in achieving their goals.

Stable structure

Although teams need to possess a stable structure, it is certainly possible for the membership to change providing that there are some continuing relationships that keep team members together and functioning as a unit.

All teams will vary in the degree to which they possess all these characteristics, but the more overt the presence of these features within the team, the more effective the team will be.

Try this at home

You may well belong to more than one team in your own organisation.

Stop and think about the following questions:

- How many identifiable teams are there within your organisation?
- Can you identify the common goals of each team?
- Are the individual members in each team aware of their common goals?
- How do your teams match up to the above criteria?

Following this analysis, it may now be apparent to you that these simple rules are often overlooked in our own work teams. In Primary Care, we frequently see colleagues following their own agenda and the goals of the organisation are not always obvious. Communication breakdown often occurs both within Primary Care teams and across them, with the majority of practices failing to take time out each day even to talk together. Perhaps your own team is closer to the dysfunctional work team in Table 4.1 rather than, say, the model of a well-organised sports team. You may also want to reflect on what the perfect size for a partnership is and compare the benefits of large and small partnerships.

Table 4.1 **Comparison of a sports team with a dysfunctional work team.**

Sports Team	Dysfunctional Work Team
Clearly defined roles for all members	Ambiguity regarding own and others' roles
Concrete measurable goal	Team goals often not apparent – differing ideas of what they are
Visible competition for the team to unite against	As much competition inside the team as outside
Has a named leader and leadership role defined	Leadership may not be obvious

Benefits of teams
Team characteristics
So that we can consider the benefits of team working, think of an outstanding team that you have worked or played in. What features made it great? They may well include some of the following factors:
• clear role definition
• clearly defined common purpose
• effective leadership
• collaborative working
• high morale
• feeling of appreciation and support
• sense of achievement and fun
• competition and rivalry uniting the team.

The need for nurturing

If all of the above features are missing we have a dysfunctional team – and most of us would have been involved in such a team at some stage of our lives. The effect on morale and self-esteem in these groups may be devastating and it is not surprising that these teams often dissolve or fragment. But in partnership, it is more than team spirit that keeps people together. There are financial ties, contracts, and many other considerations to be taken into account, all of which may deter you from leaving.

Given these potential pitfalls, it is worthwhile trying to ensure that your own team is as effective as possible. When teams function really poorly it can be extremely difficult to remedy all the faults by a process of team-building exercises, even with the help of an external facilitator. So, just as plants need feeding, teams need attention and nurturing to keep them working well.

Team vs. individual efforts

It is a common belief that teams achieve more together than the sum of the individual efforts. This can be summed up by the following acronym:

Together
Everyone
Achieves
More

But is this true, or is it just another piece of patronising business jargon? In general terms, groups produce fewer ideas in total than the individuals of those groups working separately. However, a team will often produce a better solution to a problem or a quiz than the best individual in the group; the team can evaluate ideas better and add missing data. (Also, it is often the case that 'Post It' brainstorming – when all the ideas are put down on 'Post It' notes by individuals and then evaluated – is superior to traditional brainstorming, during which quiet members of the group may feel inhibited.)

You may have participated in a 'desert survival game' or something similar, whereby individuals are asked to rank, on their own, ten items in terms of their importance in helping survivors from an air crash. The group will then discuss the importance of the ten items and produce a jointly agreed ranked list. The results are then compared to an 'expert' list and in the majority of occasions the team efforts will be superior to the average of the individual efforts.

Teams will often take riskier decisions than those of the individuals within the group. The reasons for this are unclear but may be due to a sense of shared responsibility and the desire to behave more adventurously within groups, a process of egging each other on.

Problems encountered in teams
Team vs. individual objectives

When the individuals within a team are not working towards a common goal, there are more opportunities for personal agendas to surface. These personal agendas may include making a big impression, scoring off an opponent, protecting personal interests, or making a particular alliance. Often it is not possible to satisfy all the team and individual objectives at one time and this may give rise to conflict. However, teams can also become more cohesive and drop individual concerns in times of crisis or if there is a common enemy or a competitive goal. In this situation the team becomes more productive.

'Group think'

People with similar interests, values, and personalities often form stable enduring groups. However, although heterogeneous groups tend to exhibit more conflict and take longer to form stable teams, once formed they tend to be more productive and make better decisions.

Groups that are too cohesive may become very comfortable and their commitment to harmony may cause them to succumb to *group think*. This error in decision making occurs when the group looks at too few alternatives, finds it hard to re-think a strategy that is failing, or is selective about the facts and data it considers. The group becomes blind to what is going on around it and can choose the wrong path completely. Group think can occur in the top teams of organisations and has been given as the reason for President Kennedy's involvement in the Bay of Pigs invasion.[1]

Lack of clarity

Other team problems may arise when there is a lack of clarity over the goals and purpose of the group, particularly if they are not shared by all or have been imposed. Similarly, difficulties will arise if there is confusion and blurring of the role definitions within the team or roles are allocated inappropriately.

Team formation and development

Tuckman[3] suggested that teams pass through five clearly defined stages of development, which he labelled as forming, storming, norming, performing, and adjourning (Figure 4.1). Although not all groups develop through all the stages – some get stuck in the middle, remaining inefficient and ineffective – the majority progresses through to the end. This may be a slow process, but it appears to be a necessary and inescapable route for the development of a functional team.

Forming

Forming describes the stage when the group comes together initially. Everyone is busy finding out about each other's attitudes and backgrounds and establishing ground rules. People tend to be polite and true feelings are often withheld due to a fear of upsetting others or giving the wrong impression. There is limited group identity and a strong dependence on the leader to provide direction and remove uncertainty. This stage has been likened to two dogs meeting for the first time and checking each other out before they play; the 'sniffing' stage.

Storming

Storming describes the conflict stage in the group's life and can be a painful and uncomfortable experience. Members bid for control and power and try to sort out what each of them, individually and as a group, wants out of the group process. Individuals reveal their personal goals and interpersonal hostility may be generated when the differences in goals become clear. Although it is the toughest stage it is also the most important, as decision-making processes and mechanisms for control and influence are formulated that are crucial to the effective functioning of the team. At this stage individuals may express strong opinions, challenge the ideas of others, and challenge leadership and authority. There may be complete withdrawal by some and a full expression of emotions by others. It has been likened to adolescence and many teams do not make it through this stage.

Norming

Norming refers to the cohesion that emerges where the group dynamic changes from competition to collaboration and members develop closer relationships and camaraderie. The group establishes rules and norms of behaviour, roles are allocated, and decision-making processes are decided upon. Roles may become more fluid as the group tries to use each other's skills to achieve the best results. There is tolerance for each other's strengths and weaknesses and high levels of trust within the team.

Performing

In the *performing* stage there is mutual acceptance, the group is mature and concerned with getting the job done and accomplishing objectives. There can be an intense level of loyalty and a high level of openness and trust. In terms of personal relationships, interdependence becomes a feature whereby members are equally happy working alone or in sub-groups. Such levels of autonomy require a delegating style of leadership.

Adjourning

Recognising that not all teams last forever, the final stage is termed *adjourning*. This is the disbanding stage and the reason for this may be that the task has been completed or the team disintegrates as other members leave.

Groups should be given the space to go through the various stages with no attempt to try to bypass any. An effective group leader will recognise the dynamics at each stage and adapt his or her style to the needs of the individuals whilst carrying out the task and helping the group through the *storming* phase to reach productivity and cohesion.

To illustrate these stages in the context of Primary Care, imagine that you have just created a team of individuals charged with implementing the new

Figure 4.1 **Stages of group development**

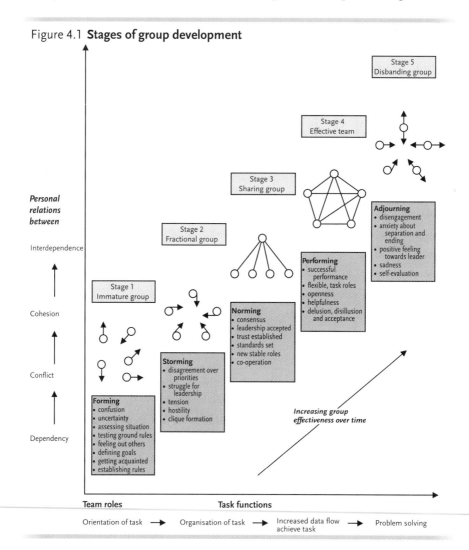

GMS Contract in your practice. At first, the team checks each other out, watching to see who comes up with the best ideas, whose suggestions are most widely accepted, and who appears to take charge (*forming*). Then as individuals struggle to get their opinions heard and gain influence over each other you may witness a battle over control of the group and some members may get upset or become unco-operative (*storming*). Once this is resolved, the group should emerge with a clear group leader, agreed objectives, and a plan for implementation that everyone owns. At this stage the group will be highly co-operative and harmonious and do things together such as meeting over lunch (*norming*). It is now possible for the plan to be implemented, the data to be collected, and goals and targets met (*performing*). Once the objectives are achieved there will be no further need for this particular group and they will *adjourn*.

Belbin

Within a team some individuals will show a consistent preference for certain behaviours and not for others. This set of behaviours may lead them to be seen as playing a particular role within the team. A popular and widely used framework for understanding roles within a group was developed by Meredith Belbin[5] in the late 1970s following lengthy research. Belbin discovered that the best teams were not necessarily those composed of the brightest individuals and concluded that there are nine team roles that are needed for a fully effective team. Each team role is listed in Table 4.2. (Note that the *specialist* role is often omitted, as Belbin added it in the 1990s.)

Belbin argued that in an ideal team all the roles are represented and that the roles that people prefer can be predicted through a team role questionnaire that he devised. Since many effective teams often comprise fewer than nine individuals, each member may comfortably perform more than one role. Belbin's framework is frequently used in Primary Care, both in practice teams and on day-release courses.

Although it appears to give some helpful insight into team roles and functions, as a result of its popularity, Belbin's theory has been extensively researched and has received considerable criticism. The team role questionnaire is based on self-reporting and as these self-perceptions are not always accurate, its reliability is questionable. As such it would be a poor basis on which to select team members, which has previously been one of its uses. The questions are also vague and inconsistent and from a research point of view, it has proved an unreliable tool. Despite this contrary evidence, his role descriptions and questionnaire continue to be a popular method for creating and analysing teams.

Table 4.2 **Belbin's team roles.**

Belbin Role Type	Team Role Contribution	Allowable Weaknesses
PLANT	Creative, imaginative, unorthodox. Solves difficult problems.	Ignores details. Too pre-occupied to communicate effectively.
CO-ORDINATOR	Mature, confident, a good chairperson. Clarifies goals, promotes decision making, delegates well.	Can be seen as manipulative. Delegates personal work.
MONITOR EVALUATOR	Sober, strategic, and discerning. Sees all options. Judges accurately.	Lacks drive and ability to inspire others. May be over-critical.
IMPLEMENTER	Disciplined, reliable, conservative, and efficient. Turns ideas into practical actions.	Somewhat inflexible. Slow to respond to new possibilities.
COMPLETER FINISHER	Painstaking, conscientious, anxious. Searches out errors and omissions. Delivers on time.	Inclined to worry unduly. Reluctant to delegate.
RESOURCE INVESTIGATOR	Extrovert, enthusiastic, communicative. Explores opportunities. Develops contacts.	Over-optimistic. Loses interest once initial enthusiasm has passed.
SHAPER	Challenging, dynamic, thrives on pressure. Has the drive and courage to overcome obstacles.	Can provoke others and hurt people's feelings.
TEAMWORKER	Co-operative, mild, perceptive, and diplomatic. Listens, builds, averts friction, calms the waters	Indecisive in crunch situations. Can be easily influenced.
SPECIALIST	Single-minded, self-starting, dedicated. Provides knowledge and skills in rare supply.	Contributes only on a narrow front. Dwells on technicalities. Overlooks the big picture.

Myers–Briggs

A more reliable method of defining team roles, and one that is increasingly used in organisations for team building, is the Myers–Briggs Type Indicator (MBTI). The MBTI identifies 16 possible personality types, each with a four-letter descriptor, taking one letter from each of the following pairs:

E or I	Extraversion or Introversion	*Indicates the way we are energised*
S or N	Sensing or iNtuition	*Indicates how we process information*
T or F	Thinking or Feeling	*Indicates how we make decisions*
J or P	Judging or Perceiving	*Indicates how we live our lives*

A full description of the MBTI preferences is found in Chapter 12.

Myers–Briggs is a powerful and empowering tool. As a team member you can use *type preferences* to understand yourself better and appreciate how you behave in a group setting. You can also use your knowledge of type to understand your team mates and the contributions they make to the team. This understanding can help you appreciate the differences between team members, which can lead to better function and less conflict. There is no such thing as a bad type, all 16 have their strengths and areas for development.

The more similar the types on a team are, the sooner the team members will understand each other; the more different they are, the slower the understanding. Groups with high similarity will reach decisions more quickly but are more likely to make errors owing to inadequate representation of all viewpoints (see 'Group think', page 42). Groups with many different types may reach their decisions more slowly but may well make more effective decisions because they cover all angles.

The MBTI can help team members by:
- identifying team strengths and weaknesses
- clarifying team behaviour
- matching task assignments with team members according to their type
- supplying a framework for team members to understand and handle conflict
- helping individuals to use differences for effective problem solving and decision making.

Team members who are opposites on all four preferences may have difficulty reaching an understanding, whereas members who share at least two preferences may act as translators. Teams with very similar types may be successful if they bring in external resources to complement their deficiencies. The person who is the only representative of a preference may be seen as different, such as the only introvert or the only feeler, but these differences need to be appreciated and their contributions valued. It has been shown that teams that appreciate type and differences may experience less conflict.

Team building

> ...At the away day the practice manager, Karen, divides the workforce up into small teams of five. Each team has one doctor and a mix of reception staff and nurses, carefully selected to reflect a balance of views and styles. The task is to analyse the audit of house calls and suggest creative solutions to the overwhelming visit load, which involves the whole primary health care team. Karen suggests that they brainstorm their ideas first on Post It notes and then discuss them in their groups. She offers champagne to the team with the best solutions.

Purpose of team building

The purpose of team building is to assist people who work together to function more effectively as a team and to help the team to work more effectively as a whole. Effective team building is concerned with the following functions:
- improving performance and results
- making better use of team and individual strengths; not concentrating on weaknesses
- resolving team problems.

Team and personal issues

Team problems are often attributed to personality clashes between team members, but these could be secondary to problems with goals, roles, and processes. Box 4.1 shows a hierarchy of team issues developed by Moxon.[6] Working through this hierarchy in descending order (from goals to relationships) can offer a safe strategy for team building, since it allows the team initially to discuss less personal issues and to clarify any problems with goals, roles, and processes. Personal issues can then be tackled in an atmosphere of trust, openness, and safety. Following through this hierarchy should, therefore, ensure that team building is a non-threatening exercise.

Team-building exercises

Team building should be a regular exercise for both new and existing teams. It is far less likely to be effective when the team is on the point of anger, distrust, and likely dissolution. It is analogous to a car needing regular servicing and oil checks to prevent the engine being ruined.

Team facilitation is not usually needed in a functional team, but if feelings are too deep-seated then it may be essential to receive feedback from someone neutral. Once interpersonal strain is out of the way then the stage is set for teams to learn to solve their own problems effectively. This does not take place

---

Box 4.1 **Hierarchy of team issues.**

Problems with goals
- Do people understand and accept the team's primary task?
- What are the team's priority objectives? Do all agree?
- How are conflicts in priorities handled?

Problems with roles
- What do team members expect of each other?
- Have these expectations been shared? Do they match?
- Do individual objectives fit in with the team's overall objectives?
- Are there areas of duplication or overlap between team roles that could be duplicated?

Problems with processes
- How are decisions taken? Are authority levels clear?
- Are the communication processes across the team working?
- Are structures, content, and processes in meetings effective?
- How are problems and conflicts resolved?
- How is activity co-ordinated? Are reporting procedures understood and adhered to?

Problems with relationships
- How do team members treat and feel about each other?
- Are people's individual needs recognised and respected?
- Does the team climate allow for open debate and sharing of concerns?
- Do the team and leader encourage feedback on team and individual performance?

---

overnight and is unlikely to follow a one-time exercise during a few days away from the organisation. Considering the great impact that effective teams have on organisational function, time given to build them is well spent.

Team building aims to create an ethos of openness and trust so that real problems and issues may be identified and tackled – going beyond the symptoms to the underlying cause. Some techniques used to build high levels of interpersonal trust may seem unorthodox. It is not uncommon for many team-building exercises to put group members into highly challenging real-life situations such as white water rafting. Such exercises are metaphors for how teams may have to pull together to meet their job challenges. There are, however, much cheaper alternatives and books on team-building exercises are readily available.[6]

Try this at home

Using hierarchy of team issues as a framework, and taking each point at a time, how does your own work team measure up to all the issues raised?

References

1.   Handy C. *Understanding Organisations*. London: Penguin, 1976.
2.   Maslow A. *Motivation and Personality*. New York: Harper and Row, 1954.
3.   Tuckman B. *Development sequences in small groups*. Psychological Bulletin 1965; 63(6).
4.   Huczynski A, Buchanan D. *Organisational Behaviour*. Harlow, Prentice Hall International, 1985.
5.   Belbin RM. *The Coming Shape of Organisations*. Oxford: Butterworth-Heinemann, 1996.
6.   Moxon P. *Building a Better Team*. Aldershot: Gower Publishing, 1993.

Further reading

Briggs Myers I, Myers PB. *Gifts Differing: understanding personality type*. Palo Alto, CA: Davis-Black, 1995.

Chapter 5

Motivation

Fraser Macfarlane

 KEY MESSAGES

- Motivation is that particular driving force within individuals by which they attempt to achieve a particular goal in order to fulfil some need or expectation.
- Individuals have a variety of changing, and often competing, needs and expectations that they seek to satisfy in a number of ways.
- There are many competing theories that attempt to explain motivation suggesting a range of motives influencing people's behaviour at work.
- Understanding the theory of motivation will help managing practitioners understand how best to motivate staff to work willingly and effectively.
- Understanding motivation will provide practitioners with useful insights into the work and career choices that they and their staff have made.

What is motivation?

Large chunks of social psychology research are devoted to answering questions about motivation in the workplace. Hunt asks a number of questions about work.[1] Why do some work so hard while others appear to coast along? Why do two people have such different rates of output? Why do some like highly structured jobs while others want freedom and independence? What makes some satisfied and happy while others seem unhappy? Why do some work alone and others spend all their time in groups? Why are some people motivated by money while others are almost unaffected by monetary rewards?

The study of motivation is concerned with 'why do people do what they do'.[2] There are four common characteristics:

1. It is an individual phenomenon – every person is unique and all the major theories of motivation allow this uniqueness to be identified and explored.

2. It is usually described as intentional. That is, it is assumed to be under the worker's control, and behaviours that are influenced by motivation, such as effort expended, are seen as actions of choice.
3. It is multifaceted. The two most important dimensions are: (i) what gets people activated (arousal); and (ii) the level of activation/arousal.
4. The purpose of motivational theories is to predict behaviour. Motivation is not the behaviour itself, and it is not performance. Motivation concerns action, and the internal and external forces that influence a person's choice of action.

Motivation and behaviour at work

The underlying concept of motivation is that of a driving force within individuals by which they seek to achieve some goal in order to fulfil some need or expectation. Why do GP registrars study for their MRCGP exams? Why do some GPs do their own out-of-hours cover? Why do some female GPs continue to work full-time when they have young children, while others reduce their hours drastically?

People's behaviour is determined by what motivates them. According to motivation theory, their performance is a product both of ability level and motivation.

> At a practice meeting, the partners of the Etchingham Park Surgery are exploring ways of further motivating their staff. The practice employs over 20 staff and is recognised locally as providing a good level of services for patients. The partners feel that most staff work well, but they are concerned that they must keep them motivated to meet the challenges of the new National Health Service. Among the motivators that are discussed are: pay rises, bonuses, fringe benefits, improved working environment, flexible working hours, more frequent staff appraisal, better access to training and development, and provision of free tea and coffee facilities.
>
> What factors should the partners take into account when making this decision? How should they decide which motivators will suit which staff?

In the example above, the partners are discussing the needs and expectations of staff. Motivation theory not only helps us to identify what we need from work but also how we can be better managers of staff. If you ask people what motivates them to go to work, the commonest answer would probably be 'To earn enough money to live'. Most people's fantasies implicitly assume that if they won the lottery tomorrow, they would immediately hand in their notice or put their business up for sale. But financial remuneration is only one of the rewards of being a member of the workforce – and occupational psychologists tell us that it is not even the most important one. Other benefits of employment include the acquisition of both an individual and a social identity, and the opportunity to interact with others in a structured and purposeful way. Since we are social animals, such interaction is essential for psychological health.

As anyone who has been unemployed knows, work maintains an individual's status and self-respect, structures the passage of time, helps ward off depressing thoughts and feelings, provides scope for personal achievement, and tests and affirms our personal competences. In addition to an overtime bonus or perform-ance-related pay, work beyond the call of duty may provide (or be perceived to provide) a boost to flagging self-esteem, higher status among one's peers, better promotion prospects, and less time to think about or confront issues in one's personal life. It seems that a range of different factors motivate us to go to work. As a starting point, the following is a useful, broad, three-fold classification for the motivation to work:

1. Extrinsic rewards – such as pay, fringe benefits, pension rights, material goods, and security. This is an *instrumental* orientation to work – work is a means to an end.
2. Intrinsic satisfaction – derived from the nature of work itself, interest in the job, and personal growth and development. This is known as a *personal* orientation to work.
3. Social relationships – such as friendship, group working, and the desire for affiliation, status, and dependency. This is known as a *relational* orientation to work and is concerned with 'other people'.

There are many competing theories that attempt to explain the nature of motivation, all of which help to explain the behaviour of certain people at certain times. However, the search for a generalised theory of motivation at work appears to be in vain. The usual approach to the study of motivation is through an understanding of internal cognitive processes – that is, what people feel and how they think.

The different theories of motivation are usually divided into two contrasting approaches: content theories and process theories. Content theories attempt to explain those specific things that actually motivate the individuals at work. These theories are concerned with identifying people's needs and their relative strengths, and the goals they pursue in order to satisfy these needs. Process theories attempt to identify the relationship among the dynamic variables that make up motivation. These theories are concerned more with how behaviour is initiated, directed, and sustained. Process theories place emphasis on the actual process of motivation. The main theories of motivation are discussed below.

Content theories of motivation

Maslow's hierarchy of needs

One model of motivation that has gained a lot of attention, but not complete acceptance, is that put forward by Abraham Maslow.[3] Scholars of philosophy may recognise that many of Maslow's ideas are similar to those of Aristotle 2000 years earlier! Maslow's theory argues that individuals are motivated to satisfy a number of different kinds of needs, some of which are more powerful, or *prepotent*, than others. The term *prepotency* refers to the idea that some needs are felt as being more pressing than others. Maslow argues that until these most pressing needs are satisfied, other needs have little effect on an individual's behaviour. We satisfy the most prepotent needs first and then progress to the less pressing ones. As one need becomes satisfied, and therefore less important to us, other needs loom up and become motivators of our behaviour.

Maslow represents this prepotency of needs as a hierarchy. The most prepotent needs are shown at the bottom of the ladder, with prepotency decreasing as one progresses upwards.

Figure 5.1 **Maslow's hierarchy of needs**

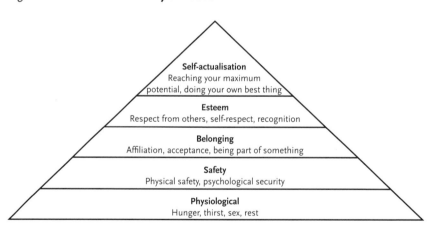

Maslow's model does not claim that individuals experience only one type of need at a time. Medical students spend much of their time learning new knowledge and skills and could be said to be motivated by self-actualisation. However, the same people, once qualified and working as junior doctors, experience sleep deprivation, challenging work conditions, and seem to live to work, eat, and sleep. The thought of self-actualisation through studying for postgraduate exams then has a lower impact than physiological needs. In fact, we probably experience all levels of needs all the time, but to varying degrees.

Similarly, in almost all organisational settings, individuals juggle their needs for security – 'Do I feel safe working here with the level of physical and verbal abuse that we get?' – with needs for esteem – 'If I do what is demanded by the job, how will my peers see me, and how will I see myself?' Given a situation where management is demanding a certain level of performance, but where group norms are to produce below these levels, all these issues are experienced. The order in which Maslow has set up the needs does not necessarily reflect their prepotence for every individual. Some people may have such a high need for esteem that they are able to subordinate their needs for safety or their physiological or belonging needs to these. The hero as GP springs to mind: 'I give all of my patients my mobile phone number and will visit them at any time, even if I am on holiday.' There is little concern for safety or physical comfort as the hero rushes forward.

Maslow asserts that once a need is satisfied it is no longer a motivator – until it re-emerges. Food is a poor motivator after a meal but can serve as a powerful motivator for hungry doctors emerging from a busy surgery, as every drug representative knows! The point in this is clear for management. If management placed emphasis on needs that have not been satisfied, employees would be more likely to be motivated towards achieving the goals of the organisation. Human behaviour, then, is primarily directed towards unsatisfied needs.

> The partners of the Etchingham Park Surgery have identified that staff seem to work in isolation and have no sense of team spirit. The partners have always put quality of patient care as a high priority and would like to explore ways of motivating staff to deliver better patient services. In discussion with staff, the partners feel that the practice has an excellent work environment and that individuals have good opportunities for personal development. Staff also recognise that they are rewarded, financially, in line with other local workers.
>
> What activities could the practice undertake that would improve team working and improve clinical care?

Frederick Herzberg's dual-factor theory

Frederick Herzberg and his associates began their research into motivation during the 1950s, examining the models and assumptions of Maslow and others.[4] The original study consisted of interviews with 203 accountants and engineers, where participants were asked to relate times when they had felt exceptionally good or exceptionally bad about their present job or any previous jobs.

On the basis of his fieldwork, he concluded that:

- There are two types of motivational factors, one type that results in satisfaction with the job, and the other that merely prevents dissatisfaction. The two types are quite separate and distinct from one another. Herzberg called the features that result in job satisfaction, *motivators* and those that simply prevented dissatisfaction, *hygiene factors.*
- The factors that lead to job satisfaction (the motivators) are: achievement, recognition, work itself, responsibility, and advancement.
- The factors that may prevent dissatisfaction (the hygiene factors) are: company policy and administration, working conditions, supervision, interpersonal relations, money, status, and security.

Motivators are those things that allow for psychological growth and development on the job. They are closely related to the concept of self-actualisation, involving a challenge, an opportunity to extend oneself to the fullest, to taste the pleasure of accomplishment, to be recognised as having done something worthwhile. Hygiene factors, if applied effectively, can at best prevent dissatisfaction: if overlooked, they can result in negative feelings about the job.

Herzberg goes further than Maslow, cutting the hierarchy off near the top and maintaining that motivation results only from some elements of esteem needs and self-actualisation.

David McClelland – the need for achievement

Many medical students take the role of the 'high achiever' at school, gaining excellent A-level results. A number of these medical students will go on to be high achieving consultants and GPs at the forefront of service development, medical politics, and service delivery. Is there a link between this need to achieve and the type of person who becomes a doctor? Could achievement be a motivator for some people? David McClelland thought so and unearthed some empirical evidence to support the view.[5] McClelland's work originated from investigations into the relationship between hunger needs and the extent to which imagery of food dominated thought processes. From subsequent research he identified four main arousal-based and socially developed motives:

1. The achievement motive.
2. The power motive.
3. The affiliative motives.
4. The avoidance motives.

The first three motives correspond, roughly, to Maslow's self-actualisation, esteem, and belonging needs. Although the relative intensity of these motives varies between individuals, the one single motivating factor that has received the most attention in terms of research is the need for achievement (*n-ach*). As a result, we know more about n-ach than any other motivational factor.

Individuals with a high n-ach have a number of distinctive characteristics that separate them from their peers. First of all, they like situations where they can take personal responsibility for finding solutions to problems, a situation that most GPs find themselves in every day. The important thing, for them, is that the outcome is the result of their own skill and effort; this allows them to gain personal satisfaction from their achievements. They do not like situations where they are not in control.

A second characteristic of high n-ach people is that they like to set moderately high goals for themselves. These goals are neither so low that they can be achieved with little challenge, nor so high that they are impossible. High n-ach individuals prefer goals that require all-out effort and the exercise of all their abilities. Rather than working to live, they live to work – being successful as a doctor is the be-all and end-all. Success is often achieved despite the working environment rather than because of it.

A third distinctive characteristic of high achievers is that they want concrete feedback on their performance. Only certain types of jobs provide this kind of feedback, however, and so some kinds of jobs are unattractive to high achievers. For instance, teachers receive only imprecise, hazy feedback as to the effectiveness of their efforts, while production managers have a daily output chart to look at with either joy or disappointment. The question is, do GPs and other managing practitioners receive adequate feedback on their performance from the people that matter?

If McClelland is right, how can we ensure that high achieving GPs are motivated? We can allow them to take responsibility for their own actions, within a national framework. We should minimise bureaucratic, day-to-day, interventions of managers and politicians. We should let GPs set their own challenging goals and ensure that they get feedback on their performance, particularly from patients and colleagues. In reality does this happen? That is for you to decide!

Process theories of motivation

The second approach to understanding motivation involves looking at how the process works rather than simply concentrating on what motivates an individual. Social psychologists have attempted to identify the relationships among the dynamic variables that make up motivation and what is required to influence behaviour and actions. By having a better understanding of this process, it is hoped that we will gain insights into what stimulates people to work harder, perhaps without gaining greater job satisfaction.

Expectancy theories

The first group of process theories that were developed were the expectancy theories of Vroom[6], and Porter and Lawler.[7] The underlying basis of these is that people are influenced by the expected results of their actions. Motivation is a function of the relationship between:

- effort expended and perceived level of performance; and
- the expectation that rewards (desired outcomes) will be related to performance.

There must also be:

- the expectation that rewards (desired outcomes) are available.

Vroom has challenged the assertion of the human relationists that job satisfaction leads to increased productivity (the 'contented cow' approach to management). The assumption is that if management keeps employees happy, they will respond by increasing productivity. For Vroom, satisfied needs do not motivate people and hygiene needs simply keep employees quiet for a time. For an individual to be motivated to perform a certain task, he or she must expect that completion of the task will lead to achievement of his or her goals. The task is not necessarily the goal itself but is often the means of goal attainment (*instrumentality*). For example, if I work hard and get monetary rewards (means), I will be able to afford a nice house (ends).

Performance therefore depends upon the perceived expectation regarding effort expended and achieving the desired outcome. An administrator's desire to be promoted to practice manager will result in high performance only if the person really expects that this will lead to promotion. If, however, the administrator believes promotion to be based solely on age and length of service, there is no motivation to achieve high performance. A person's behaviour reflects a conscious choice based on a comparative evaluation of alternative behaviours. The choice of behaviour is based on the expectancy of the most favourable consequences.

Vroom's model was based on three key variables: *valence, instrumentality* (goal attainment), and *expectancy*. The theory is founded on the idea that people prefer certain outcomes from their behaviour over others. They anticipate feelings of satisfaction should the preferred outcome be achieved. Why does a GP do all of their own out-of-hours duties? Not because they enjoy it but because it gives them satisfaction to know that they have undertaken it. Ask any marathon runner – do they enjoy running 26 miles or is it the satisfaction they get once they have finished?

The feeling about specific outcomes is termed *valence*. This is the attractiveness of, or preference for, a particular outcome to the individual; that is, the anticipated satisfaction. Vroom distinguishes valence from value. A person may desire an object but then gain little satisfaction from obtaining it. Alternatively, a person may strive to avoid an object but finds, subsequently, that it provides satisfaction – out-of-hours duties, for example.

When a person chooses between alternative behaviours that have uncertain outcomes, the choice is affected not only by the preference for a particular outcome, but also by the probability that such an outcome will be achieved: 'Will I be able to function during the day if I undertake all of my own out-of-hours commitments?' People develop a perception of the degree of probability that the choice of a particular action will actually lead to the desired outcome, known as *expectancy*. The combination of valence and expectancy determines the person's motivation for a given form of behaviour. This is the motivational force. Instrumentality describes the degree of linkage between performance-related outcomes generated by initial effort and second level, needs-related outcomes of high valency. A simplified model is shown in Figure 5.2.

Figure 5.2 **Expectancy theory of motivation**

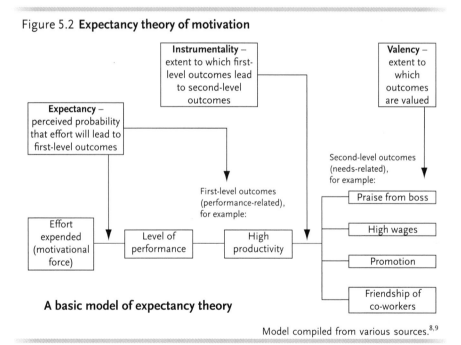

A basic model of expectancy theory

Model compiled from various sources.[8,9]

Vroom's expectancy/valence theory has been further developed by Porter and Lawler. Their model goes beyond motivational force and considers performance as a whole. They point out that effort expended (motivational force) does not lead directly to performance. It is mediated by individual abilities and traits, and by the person's role perceptions. They also introduce rewards as an intervening variable.

> *Dr Pink is a senior partner in a large rural practice. She knows that her practice nurse, Ms Blue, is capable but under-confident, when it comes to running the diabetes clinic. In particular, Ms Blue finds it difficult to deal with challenging patients and feels that she does not have the skills to manage the clinic without constant input from the GPs. How should Dr Pink motivate Ms Blue to take on more responsibility in this clinic? She knows that Ms Blue could do it, if only she were more confident.*

Implications of expectancy theories for managers

Expectancy theory seems to work intuitively, but how can it be used by GPs and others to motivate their colleagues and staff? It is in its application that managers can benefit by giving attention to a number of factors:

- Use rewards appropriate in terms of individual performance – outcomes with high valence should be used as an incentive for improved performance. Identify, by knowing your staff, what outcomes from the job they value.
- Attempt to establish clear relationships between effort-performance and rewards, as perceived by the individual. Be clear about what people are responsible for and link rewards closely to success.
- Establish clear procedures for the evaluation of individual levels of performance. Establish effective supervision and appraisal systems.
- Pay attention to intervening variables such as abilities and traits, role perceptions, organisational procedures, and support facilities, which, although not necessarily direct motivation factors, may still affect performance. Ensure that people have the skills to do the job and that they aren't prevented from doing so by outside organisational factors.
- Agree clear objectives for all staff.
- Provide feedback on performance in a clear, objective, structured way. This can be through processes such as appraisal, supervision, and audit.
- Minimise undesirable outcomes that may be perceived to result from a high level of performance, such as industrial accidents, sanctions from co-workers, short-time working, or layoffs. Make sure that you don't penalise good performance.

Better motivation, better management

Despite the largely theoretical nature of the motivation literature, it provides some useful insights into why people behave in particular ways. It also provides a toolkit for practitioners to motivate their colleagues and staff. The choice of task and reward for individuals is key in all of the process. If people understand the task, feel that they are able to be successful, and value the outcome or reward, then they are more likely to be motivated to try. As managers, therefore, we should think clearly about what we ask staff to do, find ways of giving them feedback, and ensure that they have the necessary skills and tools to be successful.

Try this at home

The motivation questionnaire at the end of this chapter has been designed to provide some insights into what you might look for at work. Once you have tried it, why not give it to a colleague and see what motivates them?

N.B. This questionnaire has not been formally validated and is intended for interest only.

References

1. Hunt J. *Managing People at Work*. Maidenhead: McGraw-Hill, 1986.
2. Pate LE. Understanding human behaviour. *Management Decisions* 1998; **26**: 58–64.
3. Maslow AH. A theory of human motivation. *Psychological Review* 1943; **50**: 370–396.
4. Herzberg F, Mausner B, Synderman BB. *The Motivation to Work*. London: Chapman Hall, 1959.
5. McClelland DC. *Human Motivation*. Cambridge: Cambridge University Press, 1988.
6. Vroom VH. *Work and Motivation*. New York: Wiley, 1964.
7. Porter LW, Lawler EE. *Managerial Attitudes and Performance*. London: Irwin, 1968.
8. Handy CB. *Understanding Organisations*. London: Penguin, 1993.
9. Mullins LJ. *Management and Organisational Behaviour*. Harlow: Prentice Hall, 1999.

Further reading

Handy CB. *Understanding Organisations*. London: Penguin, 1993.

Motivation Questionnaire

Part one: Mark with 10 points (each) the *four* items that you would look for first in your ideal job (your present job or your next job); and then mark with 4 points (each) the next *four*.

		Score
A1	Allowed to set one's own goals	
A2	Stimulating, varied work	
A3	Full, productive use of time	
A4	Working with good colleagues	
A5	Good economic rewards	
A6	Job security	
A7	Chances to be creative	
A8	Physically active work	
A9	A good boss who shows equitable leadership	
A10	Responsibility	
A11	Using one's full range of skills	
A12	Serving others	
A13	Pay is sufficient to provide a decent lifestyle	
A14	Chance of promotion and a good career structure	
A15	Easy work	
A16	Involvement in change	
A17	Good hours that don't interfere with life outside work	
A18	Difficult, challenging work	
A19	Authority to make decisions	
A20	Opportunities to travel	
A21	Good range of social activities	
A22	It gives me status in society and among my friends	
A23	Good feedback on my performance	
A24	Chance to learn, develop, and grow	

Questionnaire developed by Fraser Macfarlane.

Motivation Questionnaire

Part two: Mark with 10 points (each) the *two* things you like least about your present job and that you feel you must avoid in future jobs: then mark with 4 points (each) the next *two* things.

		Score
B1	Poor economic rewards	
B2	Insecurity and uncertainty	
B3	Pressure and demands of the work are too hard for me	
B4	Ambitions unrealised	
B5	Too long, or inappropriate, working hours	
B6	Too closely supervised by the boss	
B7	Boring, monotonous work	
B8	Poor working environment	
B9	Unpleasant boss	
B10	Horrible colleagues	
B11	No career structure	
B12	Work doesn't fit my skills or interests	
B13	Work keeps me away from home	
B14	Dirty work environment	
B15	Poor transport facilities	
B16	Dishonesty from staff and colleagues	
B17	Not being treated as an individual	
B18	Job has no impact on society	

Continued overleaf

Motivation Questionnaire

Answer sheet

What stimulates you at work? Using the completed motivation questionnaire you will be able to calculate which of your psychological needs has most influence on your attitude to work.

Transfer your scores from the questionnaire to the table below:

Primary needs	Score	Secondary needs	Score	Higher needs	Score
A5		A4		A1	
A6		A9		A2	
A8		A12		A3	
A13		A20		A7	
A15		A21		A10	
A17		A22		A11	
B1		A23		A14	
B2		B3		A16	
B5		B9		A18	
B8		B10		A19	
B13		B16		A24	
B14		B17		B4	
B15		B18		B6	
				B7	
				B11	
				B12	
Total		Total		Total	

Motivation Questionnaire

Summary
The maximum score over all three groups of needs is 84. The thing to watch is the *difference* in your three scores. There are no good and no bad character profiles. Whatever comes out is just you!

Primary needs	for comfort, safety, security, freedom from anxiety and fear, for law and order	**Score**
Secondary needs	for belongingness and acceptance, to be respected, not to be alone, for esteem, dignity, and appreciation	**Score**
Higher needs	to practice competence, work independently, learn and grow, make decisions and be responsible for them	**Score**

Above 40 in any category represents a high score.

Chapter 6

People Problems – Problem People

Antony Americano

 KEY MESSAGES

- Grievances are an employee's opportunity to raise issues of concern in the workplace.
- There are three basic legal steps to the grievance process: the employee puts their concerns in writing, there is a meeting to discuss the grievance, the employee has the right of appeal if they are unhappy with the response.
- Bullying and harassment complaints can be dealt with under the Grievance Procedure or by a separate policy.
- Disciplinary processes should be the final resort. Steps should be taken to avoid the necessity to take formal action.
- Disciplinary issues should focus on the problem and not the person.
- There are three basic legal steps to any disciplinary procedure: advise the employee in writing of the concerns and the evidence relating to those concerns, hold a disciplinary meeting at which the employee has the right to be represented and provide and question evidence, allow the employee the right of appeal against the disciplinary decision.

Introduction

People problems in the workplace are often a result of misunderstandings, competing interests, or mismatched expectations. They can be a source of enormous anxiety for all those involved (including management) and as a result are frequently ignored or avoided and so allowed to escalate. If conflict is not identified and managed at an early stage, it can be damaging to relationships within the team, but also to external stakeholder relations. An efficient and productive approach to the management of people problems requires both clear procedures in place and the ability (and will) to handle problems in a timely and consistent manner.

This chapter is written for those not experienced in the formal aspects of managing people problems at work. It is also written bearing in mind smaller health and social care settings where formal policies and procedures are less likely to be present than in larger organisations. Its aim is to be of practical use in tackling day-to-day issues, but it is not a guide to writing policies. The Advisory, Conciliation and Arbitration Service (ACAS) website is a good starting point for this (www.acas.gov.uk). Neither is this guidance a substitute for professional or legal advice.

In the first section, we discuss grievances at work and the process for handling them. We also briefly cover the specific area of workplace bullying and harassment. In the second section, we move on to exploring the main issues surrounding disciplinary action and the important steps that should precede it.

Grievances

Grievances are an opportunity for staff to formally raise concerns about conditions, changes, or treatment they are experiencing in the workplace. A manager may feel that their position of authority is being challenged when the Grievance Procedure is used. However, a grievance provides a necessary outlet for employee concerns that might otherwise fester and lead on to poor relations, disruptive behaviour, poor performance or, ultimately, to resignation and the possibility of legal action.

It is also important to reflect that the management perspective cannot fully represent the pluralist interests at work – worker/manager, differing professional backgrounds, gender, ethnicity, and so on. The Grievance Procedure allows for opinions to be heard, alternatives to be found, and managerial or organisational mistakes and omissions to be addressed and learnt from. It may even generate better ideas and new options that will be of benefit to all.

Managing formal grievances

It might be argued that it is better to manage grievances outside of formal procedures through regular discussion and dialogue, and you would be right. An open approach to management, consultation, and participation in the workplace will significantly reduce the need for formal grievances and avoid some of the pitfalls of formalised procedures.[1] Many issues are resolved at the informal grievance stage, which is often a discussion between an individual and their line manager. However, even in the best run organisation, this will not always be sufficient. Best human resource practice, as formalised in the Employment Act 2002, sets out a statutory minimum Grievance Procedure that must be carried out without unreasonable delay. Larger organisations may have more steps than those indicated below.

Step One: The employee puts their concerns in writing

The employee sets down in writing the nature of the grievance and sends the written complaint to the employer. He/she must inform the employer of the basis of the complaint.

Guidance. The complaint is normally sent to the line manager. Where the line manager is the object of the grievance, the complaint may be sent to another senior individual. There should be no stipulations about the format of the written grievance, so long as it is legible and meets the requirement of Step One. This should therefore encompass email, handwritten, and word processed documents.

It is possible that at this stage the grievance is unclear or unfocused. This is not uncommon. Staff may be unable to express themselves clearly, may not have worked out specifically what is upsetting them, or may be avoiding voicing the true concern because it is sensitive. These issues should be addressed in Step Two.

Step Two: There is a meeting to discuss the grievance

The employer should invite the employee to at least one hearing at a reasonable time and place at which the grievance can be discussed. The employee should take all reasonable steps to attend. After the meeting, the employer must inform the employee about any decision and offer the employee the right of appeal.

Guidance. Remember the employee has a right to be accompanied by a colleague or Trades Union representative. Begin by ensuring that you have a shared understanding of the employee's grievance. It is unwise to assume that you already understand the problem. Even if the problem does seem clear, there is value in allowing the employee the opportunity to voice their concern.

It is also unwise to believe you know how to resolve the grievance. The best approach is to ask them what outcome they are seeking. If the outcome seems unreasonable, e.g. requesting that another colleague be dismissed, you may need to discuss the limits of action available under the Grievance Procedure.

A further meeting may be needed, where issues raised require investigating. Again, there should be no unnecessary delay in the process. When framing the decision, you should try as much as possible to acknowledge the details of the complaint without necessarily agreeing. The following are possible outcomes:

- *The organisation is at fault.* You will want to make proposals about how you will address the problem. An apology can also go a long way to restore harmony.
- *The problem exists between two or more individuals.* You will need to consider

steps to manage this. It is not possible to ask people to like each other, but it is reasonable to require them to work professionally together.

- *There is no substance to the grievance.* You should nevertheless respect the right to raise a grievance and respond in a way that will allow the individual to return to normal working with dignity.
- *The grievance is malicious.* In a small number of cases you may feel that the person raised the grievance maliciously. In an even smaller number of cases you may have evidence of this belief. If you do, you may wish to use the disciplinary procedure to deal with this as misconduct.

Finally, you should confirm your decision, and the reasons for it, in writing. This should include informing the individual of their right of appeal.

> *Elaine is a receptionist at a practice where she has worked well for five years. She raises a complaint under the Grievance Procedure because lately she feels that she is not getting support when she has to deal with difficult colleagues. Additionally, her fellow receptionist, Jill, who has been in post for less than a year, seems to enjoy more support. Elaine feels that this is all too much after five years of hard work. She already has enough to cope with as she has split up from her long-term partner.*
>
> *You are hearing the grievance. It is a medium-sized practice and although you have not been directly involved in the issues you have heard the office gossip. You know that there has been grumbling about Elaine's attitude recently. Some people now find it easier to approach Jill. You have also heard on the grapevine that Elaine has split from her boyfriend.*
>
> *How will you plan for the meeting? How will you commence the grievance discussion? Where are the potential bear traps?*

Step Three: The employee has the right of appeal

If the employee considers that the grievance has not been satisfactorily re-solved, he/she should inform the employer that they wish to appeal against the employer's decision or failure to make a decision. The employer should arrange a meeting to discuss the appeal. After the meeting, the employer's final decision should be communicated to the employee.

Guidance. Wherever possible a more senior manager than the one who made the original decision should carry out the appeal. The employee should be advised of their right to be represented by a colleague or Trades Union representative.

It is important to explore with the employee where they feel their grievance has not been satisfactorily resolved and go through the evidence again. The manager who heard the original grievance may be present to explain how they came to their conclusions. The appeal decision should be communicated to the employee in writing indicating that this is the last stage of the organisation's grievance procedure.

Bullying and harassment

Bullying and harassment may be covered under the Grievance Procedure, but increasingly, especially in larger organisations, a separate policy is produced to deal with what can be a very sensitive issue and a legal minefield. Whichever approach you choose in your organisation, the complaint must be handled sensitively, bearing in mind the rights of both the complainant and the accused person.

The statutory definition of harassment in the Race Relations Act is as follows:

A person subjects another to harassment . . . where on grounds of race, ethnic or national origins, he engages in unwanted conduct which has the purpose or effect of: (a) violating that person's dignity, or (b) creating an intimidating, hostile, degrading, humiliating or offensive environment for him.

Bear in mind that according to this definition, harassment does not need to be intentional; it is sufficient that it led to the person feeling harassed. This position is moderated by the need to show that such feelings were reasonable in the circumstances. This definition is applicable to other types of harassment based on, for example, gender, sexual orientation, and disability.

Bullying has similarly been defined as:

Offensive, intimidating, malicious or insulting behaviour, an abuse or misuse of power through means intended to undermine, humiliate, denigrate or injure the recipient.[2]

Examples of bullying behaviour include: derogatory remarks, constantly undervaluing effort/knowledge, insulting or aggressive behaviour, ignoring or excluding an individual, and setting unrealistic deadlines or changing them without consultation or explanation. This list is not exhaustive. Bullying need not necessarily be face-to-face; it can be committed by letter, memo, email, or over the telephone.

Managers must:
- set a positive example by treating colleagues with dignity and respect
- set standards of acceptable behaviour for their team

- treat complaints seriously and take prompt action
- handle situations sensitively, respecting, wherever possible, the need for confidentiality.

Disciplinary action

If you work in a large organisation, it will most likely have its own disciplinary procedures. It is critical that you follow these and take advice from any human resource specialist working in your organisation. Employment Tribunals will not look favourably on an organisation that cannot follow its own procedures and standards. If you work in a small organisation, such as a general practice, then you may be one of those responsible for setting the processes for managing disciplinary action.

This advice draws on the case law established through the courts and, critically, on the ACAS Code of Practice,[3] a key document that summarises, in an easy to digest format, statutory provisions regarding discipline, supplemented by practical guidance. The Code, though not legally binding, is admissible in evidence at an Employment Tribunal and can be used to consider the question of fairness of a dismissal.

The legal context

The Employment Act 2002 introduces statutory minimum disciplinary and dismissal procedures. It requires all organisations to meet minimum standards and a failure to do so will make the disciplinary action automatically unfair. The next section explains how to comply with the Act and provides guidance based on the ACAS Code and case law.

The leading employment case on the reasonableness of a dismissal is that of Burchell.[4] This established a three-step test to consider the reasonableness of an employer's decision to dismiss for misconduct:

1. The employer must have a genuine belief in the employee's guilt. For example, it should not be a pretext for dismissal when other issues are the true concern.
2. This belief must be held on reasonable grounds. This step suggests that there must be evidence, facts, and/or informed views that support the decision and not prejudice or gossip.
3. This evidence must be based on as much investigation as is reasonable in the circumstances. This means an employer should look around and into the evidence to ensure that a rounded picture has been provided. Reasonableness is judged on the size and resources of the organisation, balanced against the serious effect of a dismissal on the individual.

> *An employee was dismissed after having admitted falsifying stock control documents. The employment tribunal found that, although dismissal was a reasonable response open to an employer in this situation, the disciplinary procedure followed was unfair as the employee's area manager had not only investigated the issue but also conducted the disciplinary hearing herself. She has also failed to consider all the circumstances. The employer appealed arguing that, since the employee had admitted the misconduct, the tribunal should only consider whether dismissal fell within the band of reasonableness. The Employment Appeals Tribunal and the Court of Appeal (more senior courts) dismissed the employer's appeal. The requirement of reasonableness involves not only the decision to dismiss but also the process by which the decision is reached.*
>
> *Whitbread plc v Hall (2001)*

Even where an employee admits misconduct, it is still important to follow the procedure, particularly where dismissal results. Consequently, a fair and detailed investigation is still required. Wherever possible separate people should carry out investigation and decision making, and alternatives to dismissal should be discussed.[5]

Pre-disciplinary stage

Disciplinary processes should be a final resort having exhausted other avenues and approaches. The following is a list of areas you should consider before starting the disciplinary procedure:

Clear rules. Ensure that the organisation has clear rules and procedures so that there can be no doubt or argument about appropriate behaviour.

Clear standards. Ensure that staff are clear about performance standards and that they receive regular feedback on their work. Appraisal is one method of ensuring that staff receive formalised feedback; another is to hold regular one-to-one meetings.

Training and development. Provide appropriate learning and development opportunities. This may be through formal courses but also through workplace learning, shadowing, and mentoring.

Highlight problems. If you see areas of concern, raise these at as early a stage as possible. This should be done constructively, addressing the problem and not the person. For example, do not tell someone that they cannot write properly.

Instead, let them know that their written communication is not of the standard required and go on to explain what this standard is.

Keep records. If you are dealing with a concern at the early stages, keep written records of the issues discussed, dates, and the support offered and response received. If someone is regularly late or absent, keep exact records of each occurrence.

Warn the individual. If after the above support there appears to be no improvement, you should warn the person, in writing, that unless you see improvement, the disciplinary procedure may need to be invoked.

Occasionally, issues of misconduct may be sufficiently severe to move straight into the disciplinary procedure. Most performance issues, however, would require a series of warnings interspaced with time to improve before dismissal could be contemplated.

> **Try this at home**
> Clear rules and standards are essential to managing performance and conduct at work. Imagine you are inducting a new employee into your workplace. What rules and standards would they need to know about and where would they find these? Are they written down, custom and practice, or third party; e.g. professional or legal standards? Are these arrangements sufficiently robust?

Handling disciplinary problems

The term 'people problems' can mislead us into focusing on the individual as the problem rather than on analysing the problem itself. This can impede early solutions and damage relationships. For example, is someone an aggressive person or are they someone frustrated by an unresolved concern? Are they a poor performer or are they someone who hasn't had adequate training? Keeping a focus on the problem rather than the person can often assist in a successful outcome, as it is usually easier to resolve a problem than to alter fundamental characteristics of an individual.

If you are taking disciplinary action there are three key steps laid down in law and these should be taken without unreasonable delay. The guidance below is based on case law and good practice.

Step One: Notify them in writing

You should advise a member of staff in writing about the nature of the disciplinary concern and provide them with details or evidence of this concern.

Guidance. Putting the disciplinary concern into words can be more complex than you might imagine. You must frame your allegations carefully, as it is damaging to the management case to introduce new or altered ones later. Consider whether you are you looking at an issue of misconduct (e.g. rude to patients, theft), capability (e.g. poor performance and attendance), or some other reason.

> *Two employees had received two final written warnings for lateness. After the second final warning, Mr Want was late on 12 out of 80 working days. The tribunal found the dismissal fair. The employer had followed the disciplinary procedure and it was reasonable to treat the absence history after the second final warning as warranting dismissal.*
>
> *Mr Hallet on the other hand had been late on 7 out of 77 working days after the final warning. On three occasions his lateness was caused by industrial action on the railways. His dismissal was considered unfair bearing in mind his substantial service and the considerable improvement that had occurred in his time keeping.*
>
> *Hallett and Want v MAT Transport Ltd (1976)*

You must provide the employee with the evidence supporting your concerns in the interest of natural justice; i.e. people have the right to know exactly what they are accused of and have the right to refute the evidence. For example, telling someone that they are regularly late for work is inadequate. On what days were they late and how late were they? Employees cannot defend themselves or offer *mitigation* against generalities. They also should know the evidence of witnesses, usually in a written statement, although it is not always necessary that they have the opportunity to question the witness in person. Nevertheless, this opportunity should only be denied for clear and important reasons.

Mitigation is information that attempts to lessen the severity of the complaint, and therefore the disciplinary action, by explaining the context in which it happened; e.g. you were rude to a patient but only after you had been severely provoked. Of course, this is still not acceptable, but at least, if the mitigation is accepted, we know that the person would not behave like this under normal circumstances.

> *Patients made complaints about a nurse's conduct when she was a sister in charge of a ward. The patients were not called as witnesses at the disciplinary hearing where she was dismissed. Her internal appeal was dismissed. A tribunal found the dismissal fair.*

> Her appeal to the Employment Appeals Tribunal, on the grounds that the dismissal was unfair because patients had not been called to give evidence at the hearing or the appeal, and that there was a breach of natural justice, was dismissed. Natural justice requires that the employee should know the accusations made against her and have an opportunity to state her case and that the internal appeal panel should act in good faith. It was not necessary that the complainants should have given evidence in person.
>
> Khanum v Mid-Glamorgan Health Authority (1979)

Step Two: Invite them to a meeting

> The employer must invite the employee to a meeting to discuss the concerns. The timing and location of the meeting must be reasonable. The member of staff can choose to be represented by either a colleague or a Trades Union representative.

Guidance. Wherever possible, the individual who has investigated and brought the disciplinary case should not be the person who decides on the outcome. This can be difficult in a small organisation, but it is nevertheless the standard for which you should strive. The requirement for reasonable notice means that an individual must have time to organise their defence and obtain representation. A minimum of five working days is advised.

Before dismissing someone, you must consider alternatives; e.g. demotion, transfer, disciplinary suspension. This should occur even if it is only to rule these out. If a warning is given you should consider how long this will be 'live'; i.e. a record kept and referred to in references or if future disciplinary concerns arise. Anything from 6–24 months is possible, but it should rarely be indefinite. If you develop your own policy, the period should be specified to ensure that individuals are treated consistently. Inconsistency can leave you open to claims of discrimination.

Figure 6.1 shows a standard format for a disciplinary meeting.

Step Three: Conduct an appeal hearing

> If an employee indicates a wish to appeal against the decision, an appeal meeting should be convened. Ideally, a manager who is more senior than the manager who conducted the disciplinary meeting should hear this.

Figure 6.1 **Outline of a disciplinary hearing**

Manager hearing the case	Investigating manager	Member of staff
Introduces everyone and their roles.		
Clarifies disciplinary purpose of meeting, allegations, and potential outcomes.		
Outlines briefly what is to follow.		
	Presents case against the employee, including witnesses if required.	
		Employee and representative can cross-question the investigating manager and any witnesses.
Additional questions to investigating manager and any witnesses.		
		With support of representative to present their defence including any witnesses.
	Cross-questions the employee and any witnesses.	
Additional questions to employee and any witnesses.		
	Summary of his/her case.	
		Summary of his/her case.
Parties asked to leave and return at a specified time. Considers information presented.		
Both parties called back to hear the decision.		
The decision should be confirmed in writing, including the right of appeal.		

Guidance. When you hear an appeal you can choose between considering only appeal points put forward by the employee or to rehear the case in its entirety. A rehearing has the advantage that it can correct earlier mistakes that might otherwise make the decision legally unfair. At a minimum, another manager at the same level as the one who made the decision can hear the appeal, but, again, it is preferable for someone more senior to be involved. The outcome of the appeal must be confirmed in writing. As above, if the appeal is against dismissal, you must consider possible alternatives before confirming the original decision.

References
1. Cropanzano R, Byrne ZS. When it's time to stop writing policies. An inquiry into procedural injustice. *Human Resource Management Review* 2001; **11**: 31–54.
2. www.acas.org.uk/publications/AL04.html (last accessed December 2003).
3. Advisory, Conciliation and Arbitration Service. *Code of Practice on Disciplinary and Grievance Procedures.* London: ACAS, 2000.
4. British Home Stores Ltd v Burchell (1978) Industrial Relations Law Review 379.
5. Industrial Relations Law Bulletin – April 2001, pp. 11–15.

Further reading
You may find the following websites useful:

Department of Trade & Industry (DTI) The government department responsible for employment legislation. The website provides a wealth of guidance notes on many issues, particularly employee relations: www.dti.gov.uk/er/index.htm.

CIPD The website of the Chartered Institute of Personnel & Development: www.cipd.co.uk.

ACAS The Advisory, Conciliation and Arbitration Service. A government-sponsored body that has the tasks of promoting good employee relations. There is an on-line learning program for developing disciplinary and grievance procedures: www.acas.gov.uk.

Bullying and harassment Some useful research and case studies on the subject: www.workplacebullying.co.uk.

A few books, too:
Advisory, Conciliation and Arbitration Service. *ACAS Handbook: discipline and grievance at work.* London: ACAS, 2003.

Jackson T. *Handling Discipline: good practice.* London: Chartered Institute of Personnel and Development, 2001.

Jackson T. *Handling Grievances: good practice.* London: Chartered Institute of Personnel and Development, 2000.

Chapter 7

Negotiation

Andrew Wilson

 KEY MESSAGES

- Go for a *win-win* outcome wherever possible.
- Consider *why* before *what* – avoid early solutions.
- Seek information and evidence.
- Be soft on the person but hard on the problem.
- Be clear about your best alternative to a negotiated agreement.

This chapter looks at what is meant by the term negotiation and the skills required to reach lasting agreements.

What is negotiation?

We all have different ideas about the meaning of the term 'negotiation'. It is often seen as the same as bartering. You are buying something in the market on holiday, you want it as cheaply as possible, the seller wants to maximise his profit. A battle of wits ensues and the resulting compromise depends on a combination of luck, bravado, and assertion. Neither of you will ever meet again, so no holds are barred!

Negotiation in a National Health Service (NHS) setting should be something different. There is often a 'win-win' outcome available, an outcome that may benefit both sides and lead to an enhanced future relationship. This requires *principled negotiation*.

Consider these three situations and the interpersonal skills required:

Given two or more parties:	
They have common aims	Requires the skills of co-operation and teamwork
Either they have different aims that are incompatible, or one has no wish to agree	Requires the skills of influencing, coercion, and persuasion, or walk away with no agreement
They have different aims but wish to reach agreement	Requires the skills of negotiation to reach a lasting agreement, or agree not to agree

The first situation is about *teamwork* and should lead to a satisfactory outcome (the reader is referred to Chapter 4 for an insight into effective team working). The second situation will often lead to *compromise*; a halfway solution where neither party is really happy with the outcome.

This chapter addresses the third situation. The aims may well be different, but it is in the interest of both sides to seek agreement. That agreement needs to last and to be compatible with an ongoing relationship. This is the win-win of *negotiation*.

Interests vs. positions

Your 'aims' or 'interests' in a negotiation represent the *why* of the negotiation. Your 'position' represents the *what*. Ultimately, any negotiation will finally be defined as *what* has been agreed, but defining *what* too early can lead to failure to agree.

> *My daughter recently passed her driving test. For the previous year her brother had become used to having sole use of our spare old car. Within 24 hours of him returning from university a fight broke out; they both wanted the car that night. The positions seemed incompatible. The two of them started on issues of fairness; he should have the car because he needed it to get to his friends and hadn't driven the thing for three months. She should have it as she had only just passed her test, and he had had sole use for a year. Then they turned to considering a compromise – tossing a coin. The loser had the car the next day but one would be unhappy. The third option approaching was to fight it out. Then they both came to their senses and looked at the question 'why'. Why did each have to have the car now? He wanted it to visit friends who lived nowhere near public transport – he wasn't interested in the driving of the car, just getting there. She had previously arranged (with her mother) for a first supervised drive on the motorway that evening. Ascertaining their interests, the 'why' factor, was all too easy. She drove him to his friends on the motorway, whilst he acted as her supervisor for her first motorway drive. Both were happy – win-win!*

Consider this next experience:

> *Proud of my training and my hard won MRCGP, I started in practice as the new, unknown GP in an affluent and demanding area. Pretty soon I had seen a series of patients who responded to my 'How can I help you?' with the statement, 'I should like you to refer me to the best specialist in*

(say) dermatology.' I felt deskilled and rather angry. Here I was, well trained in a condition that I wanted to treat, and all they wanted was a referral. It seemed as if our intentions were incompatible. However, it was really only the initial positions that were incompatible. Let's look at the underlying aims.

The patients wanted to get better. I wanted them to get better and to practice the medicine I had learnt. These, I realised were not, in fact, contradictory. I learnt to say 'Yes, no problem referring you to the best consultant, but before we decide which consultant will be best, I need to understand better what is going on. Try this cream for a week then let's review and decide who will be most suitable.' Inevitably on return, things had improved, and they no longer wanted referral – both our aims had been met.

When considering any situation try to stand back from early solutions. Think about your aims and interests, and what the aims and interests of your sparring partner might be. If you become stuck with incompatible solutions, ask them to consider their aims. I once worked for a dynamic Director of GP Education, full of ideas in the form of solutions. I learnt to say, 'And to what problem is that a solution, Patrick?'; this got us back to considering aims before solutions. Always have the 'why' ready to use when someone is rushing into solutions.

Information gathering and exchange

It always pays to find out about the other side. Ask questions and listen; try to find out where they are coming from and what their interests are. Understanding their interests may help you find an agreeable solution. More difficult is how much you disclose of your situation. If they are keen to make a fair and lasting agreement, and you will have an ongoing relationship, there may be a lot to gain by sharing your situation and interests with them. This may be the quickest way to reach a lasting agreement. However, if their motives are less than honourable, you could be putting yourself in a vulnerable position. Always gather information and listen. Giving information carries benefits and risks.

Generating options for mutual gain

If you are able to share interests with the other side then the opportunity to generate creative options opens up. You can then use your joint creative energies to brainstorm imaginative options. The aim is to find low cost/high gain options, where each party can give something of great value to the other but at little cost.

> *I was delighted to get my first choice of vocational training scheme, but it required a move and buying our first house. I had already developed distrust of the estate agent for trying to gazump us, and the words 'handy for the motorway' had meant that you could hear it night and day. However, during the negotiation we met the selling couple, and got on well. We ended up sharing information about each other over a few beers. They were selling the house to emigrate and felt stuck – they didn't know what to do with all their furniture. They would not get much for it second-hand, and couldn't take it with them. We were moving into our first house and had nothing; we would have to buy everything we needed. We soon generated a new option: we would buy the house and all its contents. We could offer more than they would ever get through a second-hand shop or newspaper, and it would cost us a fraction of the price of new or second hand purchases. The deal was very successful. They moved out with a few clothes in suitcases, we moved in and had breakfast with the milk and cornflakes they had left, using their cutlery and plates.*

In this example the option involved a high gain at low cost but required the risk of sharing information.

Managing the relationship – separate the person from the problem

So often negotiations become unstuck because the issues get mixed up with the relationships and the personalities. You won't always like the people you have to negotiate with, and vice versa – many negotiations have foundered over person-ality clashes of no relevance to the issues. The principle to follow is to separate the *person* from the *problem*, but manage both.

Make an active effort to develop a relationship with the other side. Ensure that correspondence and meetings are courteous. Avoid behaviours that might irri-tate the other side. Classic examples are immediately disagreeing after the other party speaks, or forever calling on the other side to 'be reasonable' in their negotiations, implying that their ideas are not valid as they aren't being realistic.

By managing both separately it is possible to be *soft on the person, but hard on the problem*. By keeping the issues and the relationship separate you can continue a good relationship even while discussing areas where you have very different views.

Objective evidence

Where possible seek out objective and independent information and points of reference, relevant to the issues. This is a powerful tool to ensure fair, just, and lasting agreements. A simple example might be to look at Glass's Guide to car prices before starting negotiations to buy a second-hand car, or getting an AA survey to ascertain its condition. You may be joining a new partnership and unsure of some of the norms such as starting salary, time to parity, etc; collecting information on recent local agreements of other new partners might help ground the discussions.

> Soon after starting in practice – in a rather run-down prefab in the garden of the senior partner – a prime piece of land came up for auction. Perfect for a new surgery! But the land was up for auction and there was no way we were able to bid. First we had to obtain a valuation from the district valuer, something that would take months. We found a local developer who agreed to bid for us on the informal basis that if he won, we would enter into negotiations with him to build us a new surgery. He won the auction, plans were drawn up, and then the shock – the developer's estimate was double what we could afford. Negotiations went nowhere as he insisted on his position. So we decided to show him the 'Red Book', which detailed the government's pricing of new buildings under the Cost Rent scheme. We agreed that this was objective evidence that neither side could influence. After further discussion we agreed that he would build us a surgery for the 'Red Book' costings, and subsequent negotiation would centre around the specification of the building and not its cost. We ended up with a good working relationship and a lovely new surgery.

It is always wise to look for any objective evidence around the issues you are negotiating. Are there any objective reference points or precedents?

Best alternative to a negotiated agreement (BATNA)
It is often assumed that the best outcome is an agreement, but sometimes the best outcome is *no* agreement. It is always worth considering what your alternatives are to a negotiated agreement. If these are not good, can you make them better?

Take the situation where you are keen to develop your skills in dermatology, and the local Primary Care Trust (PCT) offers you a Clinical Assistant post. This pays very poorly and wouldn't even cover your time out of practice. You may look at your alternatives – would the PCT, or another nearby Trust, be interested in your skills, and prepared to pay on a higher scale? If so, you have improved your position and may either use this information in your negotiations with the original Trust, or just opt not to negotiate and go for the better offer.

Always think about the alternatives, and how you can make them better.

Another area to think about is the other side's alternative to a negotiated agreement. This may be weak and they do not know it – would it help you to ensure that they know their alternatives are weak? In rebuilding, we had thought we were weak as we were at the mercy of the developer. However, the truth was that the developer had borrowed his money to buy the land on the back of a guarantee to the bank that he already had a buyer for the first building on the site – our surgery. If we had pulled out, he would have had financial problems – his position was also weak in that he needed us as much as we needed him!

> I used to work as a course organiser and had experienced difficulties with the quality of education provided by a local Obstetrics and Gynaecology (O&G) unit. They were very friendly consultants but saw themselves training the future O&G specialists, and not GPs. There was a little envy too, as off the record they acknowledged that the GP Senior House Officers (SHOs) were often better than their own career O&G ones. Despite our best endeavours, all attempts to improve the education failed. We had to look at our alternatives. We could remove O&G from the rotation, but it was a popular option in attracting applicants to the scheme. They saw the alternative as just taking career O&G SHOs. We felt in a weak position and so explored with the deanery their alternative to a negotiated settlement. It turned out that if they were failing to provide adequate education, they would lose not just the GP SHOs but funding for all their SHOs. We clarified this position and explained it to them. Once aware of this serious alternative we found ourselves in a new positive working relationship looking together at ways to make the education programme work.

So, considering the alternatives, both yours and theirs, is particularly important if you feel that you are in a weak position, as they may also be in a weak position. If you are both in a weak position, there may be the tendency to avoid sharing information, thus reducing the chances of generating creative solutions. Also, in this situation it may be more important than ever to use objective criteria to avoid unsatisfactory agreements. Similarly, if you both have strong alternatives, it might be hard to reach agreement and a creative solution (see Table 7.1).

Planning

Planning a negotiation is crucial to success. It is very easy to be bamboozled into an undesirable agreement by not having first planned the negotiation.

Table 7.1 **Negotiation – positions and stratregies.**

	We are weak	We are strong
They are weak	• Wide variety of possible outcomes • Likely to agree but need objective criteria to avoid unjust outcomes • May be reluctant to share information to detriment of both	• We may be happy to share info, they may be secretive
They are strong	• Are they really that strong. Can we strengthen our alternatives and see weaknesses in theirs? • Need to protect ourselves with objective criteria • They may not need an agreement, so can we find mutual interests and generate low cost/high gain options?	• High risk of no agreement, both missing out on opportunities • Should be easy to share information • Good situation to look for low cost/high gain options

Planning the process. Think about managing the relationship. How can you ensure you are 'soft on the person'? Choose amiable surroundings with refreshments. You don't have to agree at a first meeting, you may need an adjournment to reflect on progress and gain more information. If possible, make the process of negotiating co-operative. Develop the agenda and if possible, generate options together.

Planning the negotiation. Think about the negotiation using the headings in Table 7.2. What are our interests and theirs? Don't define a *bottom line*, but think of a range of acceptable solutions. Think about what you want to know from them – and what you might usefully share. Think about any creative options. Are there any sources of independent information to help ground your negotiations? What is your best alternative to a negotiated agreement? Can it be improved? What is their alternative?

Table 7.2 **Key themes in planning a negotiation.**

	Us	Them
Interests/Aims *Why?*		
Information *To share or not?*		
Find objective independent evidence		
Generating options *High gain/low cost*		
Best alternative to a negotiated agreement *How to strengthen ours? Is theirs weak?*		
Summarise and record the detail *What?*		
Manage the process *Soft on the person, hard on the problem.*	Can we co-operate on the process? Agree the agenda and generate options together Use communication skills from the consultation listening, summarising, reflecting, 'I' statements	

Making an agreement stick

It is always great to come out with an agreement, but so often it fails to come to fruition after the initial shaking of hands. The commonest reasons are these:

Misunderstandings about what has been agreed. Ensure both sides concur with what has been agreed, and write it down. Be specific. This is a time to cross the t's and dot the i's. Detail matters in making agreements stick.

The person you negotiate with does not have the authority to make the agreement. I have learnt the importance when negotiating with the PCT to ensure before a meeting that the person negotiating has the authority to make and honour an agreement.

Rackham's evidence

Ultimately, you will find that what works best for you in negotiations is personal, and hopefully by addressing the principles given above, you will find your own best strategies. A classic piece of research carried out in 1978 by Neil Rackham and John Carlisle[1] highlights behaviours that you may find helpful to adopt.

Rackham and Carlisle looked at skilled negotiators who were rated as effective by all sides, having produced lasting agreements with successful implementation. Then they observed a series of negotiations, comparing the successful negotiators with a group of average negotiators. The features exhibited (and avoided by) the skilled negotiators are shown in Box 7.1. Many of these will be familiar from your own consultations with patients.

Box 7.1 **Behaviours of skilled negotiators.**

Behaviours favoured by skilled negotiators
- Seeking information more often.
- Testing, understanding, summarising, and reflecting back.
- Concern for detail.
- Labelling contribution – starting an intervention with an indication of its nature; e.g. 'I'd like to ask you a question' or 'I'd like to make a suggestion'. Conversely, they would avoid labelling disagreements – the quickest way to stop the other side listening is to say 'I should like to disagree . . .' It is much better to give your views, and then say 'For those reasons I . . .'
- Talking about feelings using 'I' statements rather than launching accusations at the other party's behaviours; e.g. 'I am feeling uncomfortable about that . . .'
- Careful planning with a flexible agenda, thoughts on a range of options, possible common ground, and a range of outcomes; i.e. they avoid starting with a rigid bottom line.

Behaviours avoided by skilled negotiators
- Irritators; e.g. appealing to the other implying if they disagree they are unreasonable – 'Now be reasonable . . .' – the implication being that if you disagree with me you are unreasonable.
- Immediate counter proposal.
- Argument dilution – our scientific background encourages us to collect as many arguments as possible, but in negotiating if you present many arguments, the last few will be weaker and easily shot down. It is better to stick to a few, strong arguments.
- Defence-attack spiral. One party accuses the other who defends and counterattacks; the spiral starts.

Trust

Should I trust the other party? Should I distrust them? Both have risks. We seem to lack a word in English to cover absence of trust or distrust when we just don't know. One-time B movie star and American president, Ronald Reagan had a strategy in his international relations: *Trust and Verify*. By this Reagan meant, start relationships by assuming the other party will be trustworthy, but always check out the facts. If someone is being honest, they won't mind you seeing the evidence. If they assure you there is a regulation supporting their position, fine, but let's see it.

Dirty tricks

Not everyone plays fair and you may meet others who don't want to negotiate, or are only interested in pursuing their own aims. Sometimes this takes the form of *the positional bargainer* who just knows what he wants and will bully to get it. I have certainly met this problem within the NHS. Tips in dealing with these situations include:

- Don't get mad – remember *be soft on the person, but hard on the problem.*
- Use 'I' statements about how you are feeling.
- Try and build a relationship.
- Avoid rising to any provocation, respond calmly and rationally.
- Try to move the other person away from fixed positions onto interests – the 'why' questions. Ask what the other party wants to achieve and why, and share your own aims.
- Try and work co-operatively. Are there aspects of the negotiation you can co-operate on? The process of working towards an agreement, where to get objective evidence perhaps, or generating together a range of possible options?
- Protect yourself with objective criteria if possible.
- Ask for justification and sources for his 'facts'.
- Ask questions to help problem solve. Why? What if? Justification?
- Make it easy for the other party to say 'yes' without loss of face.

Summary

Principled negotiation done well is rewarding to undertake and can result in personal satisfaction and benefit for all concerned. Like consultation skills, the ability to negotiate well can be learnt. As with the consultation, theory and evidence can help, but the added active ingredient is your own reflection, both during and after live negotiations.

Try this at home

Choose a real negotiation that is coming up in your life.

Use the planning table (Table 7.2) of key negotiation themes, adding your own. Make notes before the negotiation on each of the themes. Ensure that you focus not only on seeing things from your side but also from their side. Ensure you look for any possible objective evidence in advance.

Write out your plan for managing the process of the negotiation. Where are you going to meet? Can you co-operate on any aspects such as jointly producing the agenda?

References

1.   Rackham N, Carlisle J. The effective negotiator part I: the behaviour of successful negotiators. *Journal of European Industrial Training* 1978; **2(6)**: 6–11.

Further reading

Fisher R, Ury W, Patton B. *Getting to Yes.* [2nd edn.] New York: Arrow, 1997.
Ury W. *Getting Past No.* New York: Random House, 1992.

Acknowledgement

I should like to thank Mr David Claridge, formerly of the Coverdale Organisation, and now a Consultant in Negotiation and Co-operation Skills for his inspirational teaching on the subject, which fired up my own interest and enhanced my performance in many subsequent negotiations as a result.

Chapter 8

Managing Change Effectively

Julia Oxenbury

There's nothing permanent except change.

Heraclitus (540 BC)

We are entering an age of unreason, a time when the future, in so many areas, is to be shaped by us and for us; a time when the only prediction that will hold true is that no prediction will hold true; a time, therefore, for bold imagining in private life as well as in public; for thinking the unlikely and doing the unreasonable.

Charles Handy (1989)

> **KEY MESSAGES**
> - Change is inevitable and the rate of change is increasing.
> - Slow, steady change can make you vulnerable – don't be a boiled frog!
> - Individuals and organisations need to be adaptable and adept (at change management).
> - Be sensitive to individuals' feelings in times of change – reactions to change vary.
> - For personal change, remember the sigmoid curve and don't miss the road to the future.
> - Learning organisations adapt to change faster.
> - Know how to implement, and decrease resistance to, your own innovations.

Introduction

At the time of writing this chapter my practice is in a state of minor turbulence, as we prepare ourselves for the introduction of the new GP contract and experience our first National Health Service (NHS) appraisals. Both these changes require a significant amount of personal work, which comes in addition to the day-to-day business of patient care. They are changes that will affect all practices in the country and responses will vary from practice to practice, and between individuals. Change is a constant in General Practice as well as throughout organisations and society (although it has been estimated that the rate of change for all will double every five years). What varies is the *type* of, the *reasons* for, the *ease of implementing*, the *reactions* to, and the *effects* of change. This chapter is intended to help you understand, and benefit from, the change process and enable you to implement change with good results. It will provide some change management models that should help you deal with change effectively and offers some exercises to help you place these models in context.

> **Try this at home**
> Try to list all the major changes that have impacted on your practice in the last three years.
> • Choose one that had a significant effect upon you.
> • What were the positive things about this change?
> • What were the negative or painful things about it?

Types of change
Incremental change
This is progress by evolution rather than revolution, and although after a long period one might well notice a considerable difference, incremental change has no real impact on an organisation while it is happening. This change feels safe, comfortable, and under control. It's concerned with tinkering for continuous improvement rather than anything radical. In his thought-provoking book *The Age of Unreason*,[1] Charles Handy argues that this type of change may be dangerous and to illustrate the point uses the analogy of the boiled frog. If a frog is put in cold water and the water is heated very slowly, the frog will adapt to the surrounding rise in temperature; it will become accustomed to the heat and allow itself to be boiled alive. By embracing continuous and incremental change it is possible to let our defences down and disaster in.

Discontinuous change
Discontinuous change is more fundamental, more revolutionary. It requires a mindset that will challenge existing methods and ask 'Why?'; one that will create new rules and ways of learning. Discontinuous change can be more exciting for those involved, especially those risk-takers who enjoy creating new ground rules, but it can result in traditional thinkers feeling offended and undermined as their ways are replaced. Other terms that have been used to describe this type of change include 'strategic', 'visionary', and 'transformational'. By

definition, discontinuous change has a considerable impact upon the organisation and the individuals concerned.

Degree of urgency and resistance

For both incremental and discontinuous change there are two other factors to be considered that will affect the method used to implement the change: the degree of *urgency* and *resistance*.

In General Practice, urgent changes may be required in certain circumstances, such as following a tragedy, a mistake, or a media scare. In these situations the practice needs to analyse the problem expediently, looking for causes and solutions. There will be a need for a rapid adaptation and evidence of learning from the event. Learning may be fairly superficial or take place at a deeper, more meaningful level (see *Single and double loop learning*, page 98). Change precipitated by crisis is usually viewed as a threat not an opportunity, but there is a potential for rich learning and deep change.

Resistance to change is commonly encountered in the NHS, particularly when the change is imposed (usually by the government). Often when people do not acknowledge the need for change or resent the instigators or method of instigation, they will try to block it.

Reasons for change

The need for change within an organisation or practice may be prompted by a variety of triggers, which may originate from within or without the organisation. These triggers may indicate that current arrangements, systems, practices, and procedures are no longer effective.

External triggers for change within General Practice include:
- developments in technology
- developments in treatments
- changes in patients' needs and demands
- the activities and innovations of rivals
- new legislation and government policy
- changes in contractual agreements
- changes in local policy
- changes in cultural and social values.

Internal triggers for change include:
- low morale and performance (triggering job redesign)
- new treatments and protocols
- new members of the team
- gaps in skills and knowledge base (triggering training)

- change or redesign of the building
- problem recognition or complaints
- service redesign
- peer pressure.

Reactions to change

Organisational change need not necessarily be a reactive process. We all know of innovative practices that always seem to anticipate change and are proactive in implementing novel ideas. These practices profited from first-wave fundholding and Personal Medical Services (PMS) and grasp the opportunities in new policies and redesign. It has been said that there are three types of responders to changes:

The innovators	Proactive, generate ideas, thrive on change, and believe in changing what is there.
The early adopters	Will take up new ideas and implement them, work in adaptive and flexible organisations, see opportunities.
The laggards	Last to take up new ideas, would rather others tested them out, suspicious of change and prefer the old order.

Rapid and persistent change may be the norm, but it may have a detrimental effect on the individual or organisation concerned. Toffler[2] argues that the rate of change is out of control and that society is 'doomed to a massive adaptational breakdown'. He believed that there is a limit to the amount of change an individual can tolerate and argued that 'the shattering stress and disorientation that we induce in individuals by subjecting them to too much change in too short a time is unhealthy'. He labelled this response 'future shock'.

It has also been suggested that we can react to change in the same way as we cope with a major loss or bereavement.[3] When experiencing change, people may progress through a number of different stages, firstly shock, denial, and emotional turmoil, followed by acceptance, and finally integration of new ideas and strategies. Clearly, not everybody will experience all these elements as a reaction to change, and those that do will experience different stages at different times and to different degrees. This concept, however, serves to show the profound effect that change may have on individuals when it is imposed and unwelcome.

Response to changes within Primary Care

Recent organisational changes in General Practice have been blamed for the low morale within the profession, which in turn has contributed to increasing levels of burnout and recruitment and retention problems. The term *change fatigue* has been used to describe the effect on a profession reeling from continually imposed changes to its work pattern and a top–down style of implementation. On a personal note, I remember distinctly the emotions that I experienced when fundholding was withdrawn and, as a practice, we experienced a loss of all the patient services we had worked hard for. These feelings included disbelief, anger, and disinterest in the alternative structure. This reaction affected our response as a practice to subsequent initiatives such as PMS. In reality, we missed out on an opportunity to improve our services.

Individual responses to change

Typical responses of an individual to differing levels of pressure are shown in Table 8.1. Too little pressure can cause us to become bored and unproductive, while too much causes detrimental effects on performance and health. We have all seen patients in our surgery who have suffered from extreme work stress and ceased to function adequately. We function best when we are stretched and pushing our natural limits, getting ourselves out of the comfort zone and taking on new challenges. As autonomous individuals it is best if we are in control of this process and responsible for our own development.

Table 8.1 **Pressure/performance relationship.**

Pressure level	Response	Experience	Performance
Very low	Boredom	Low levels of interest, challenge, and motivation	Low, acceptable
Low to moderate	Comfort	Interest aroused, abilities used, satisfaction and motivation	Moderate to high
Moderate to high	Stretch	Challenge, learning, development, pushing the limits	High, above expectations
High to unrealistic	Stress	Overload, failure, poor health, dysfunctional coping behaviour	Moderate to low
Extreme	Panic	Confusion, threat, loss of self-confidence, withdrawal	Low, unacceptable

The sigmoid curve

> *Eleanor is a retainee in a five-partner training practice. At a recent non-principal conference she was really excited by the session on life coaching. It makes her realise that her career has been in a bit of a rut. She seeks out her educational supervisor to ask if the practice would support her training to be a GP with a special interest in colposcopy. Although there is not currently such a post in the Primary Care Trust, she has decided to prove that there is a clinical need through local research and to produce a business case.*

Throughout our lives we all experience personal change, but how much of that change is reactive and how much proactive? Handy[4] argues that in 'the paradox of our times: by the time you know where you ought to go, it's too late to go there; or, more dramatically, if you keep on going the way you are, you will miss the road to the future'.

Figure 8.1 **The sigmoid curve**

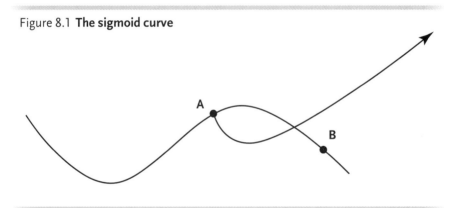

This is summed up in his concept of the sigmoid curve (see Figure 8.1). Whenever we take on a new challenge, we start tentatively, learning as we go, but it seems hard work initially as we find our way. This is represented by the initial downwards part of the curve. As we gain experience and confidence we begin to climb the second part of the curve and become more productive and effective. Inevitably, we will reach the top of the curve and begin the descent. We are now in our comfort zone, perhaps a little bored, taking things for granted and cruising. At this stage (point B) events, such as the break up of a relationship, redundancy, or a change in working practices, may occur to catapult us into another curve. Handy suggests that the time for us to change is at point A, when things seem to be going extremely well and we are close to our peak, when it would appear folly to change; this is the time to reinvent our personal strategy, be proactive, and take on a new challenge. It takes less energy and resources to change here and we restart higher up the curve with more credibility and a background of success. At point B we may already have missed our road to the future and this change is reactive.

Using the sigmoid curve as a tool for personal change can allow you to be more proactive and effective as an individual and can enhance your life and career.

Understanding organisational change

Harvey-Jones[5] commented that organisations will need to adapt or perish in the current climate, as change is one of the most pressing factors facing their managers and employees. As mentioned earlier, there is a relentless stream of pressures, both external and internal, for organisations within the NHS to adapt to political, economic, social, and technological developments. Standing still is not an option.

Learning organisations

It is said that *learning organisations* are flexible and readily adaptable and that they facilitate their staff in helping them embrace change. These are organisations in which change-oriented thinking is a habit for everybody. People in learning organisations react more quickly when their environment changes because they know how to anticipate changes that are going to occur.

The concept of the learning organisation originally derived from the work of Argyris and Schön[6] and became fashionable in the 1990s through the work of Peter Senge, whose book *The Fifth Discipline*[7] became an international best-seller. Senge argues that work needs to be more concerned with learning at all levels within the organisation and he identified five *learning disciplines* for building these learning capabilities:

Personal mastery	A commitment to continuing professional development and aspiration.
Mental models	A discipline of reflection and enquiry into the way we see and interpret things, our deeply held beliefs of how the world works.
Shared vision	A sense of commitment within a group towards a common purpose and a shared future.
Team learning	A commitment to collective thinking, learning, and action to achieve common goals.
Systems thinking	An understanding of interdependency, complexity, and the role of feedback in system development.

A change-adept organisation, therefore, has realistic goals that everyone buys into, is willing to challenge assumptions, commits to a shared vision, and works and learns as a team. Senge believed that the most important of the five 'disciplines' was *systems thinking*: understanding how complex organisations function and how they can be changed to work more effectively. According to Moss Kanter,[8] change-adept organisations show three key attributes: the imagination to innovate, the professionalism to perform, and the openness to collaborate and network. These attributes she summed up in three words: *concepts*, *competence*, and *connections*.

Organisational structure

Building a learning organisation is only possible if the culture within that organisation is suitable. Mintzberg *et al*[9] outlined the necessary cultural values to achieve the required state:

Celebrate success	Make everyone a hero when things go well. Remember that genuine praise is a powerful motivator and prove that the organisation places value on attainment.
Avoid complacency	Never sit still. Past achievements do not guarantee future success.
Tolerate mistakes	Learning organisations really do not have a blame culture. Innovation inevitably creates errors, but these are events that can be learned from and often have positive spin-offs.
Believe in human potential	Learning organisations foster personal and professional development and recognise that individuals and teams need to use their ideas and energy to achieve organisational success.
Recognise tacit knowledge	Individuals working closest to the systems often keep important information within their head. Tapping into this wealth of detail will often reveal fundamental holes within the system. This knowledge should be valued.
Encourage openness and trust	A safe environment is required to allow people to voice their ideas and concerns. Learning organisations have good communication networks that allow knowledge and views to be disseminated.
Look outward	Learning organisations network widely and share ideas and innovations with competitors.

Single and double loop learning

Argyris and Schön also described the concepts of *single loop* and *double loop* learning within an organisation (Figure 8.2). To illustrate the former, they offered the example of a thermostat controlling the heating within a room. By detecting temperature variations, it takes corrective action to maintain a constant state. What the thermostat does not do though is ask whether this was the correct temperature in the first place or whether alternative forms of heating or insulation would be necessary. In single loop learning, such values and assumptions remain unchallenged.

Figure 8.2 **Single and double loop learning**

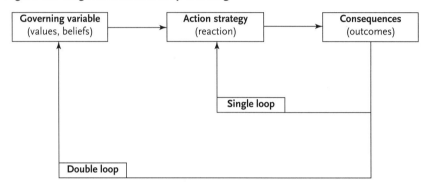

Double loop learning requires us to challenge our beliefs rather than to blindly accept them and work within their confines. The rationale for doing things in certain ways is questioned and involves constantly asking the question 'Why?'. The whole system is analysed and adapted, not just cause and effect. The result is deeper and more effective change.

To illustrate single loop and double loop learning in practice we can use the example of a *significant event analysis* involving a near miss, when a mistake in the repeat prescribing system results in a patient being issued with an incorrect drug. Single loop learning would result in remedying of the error on the computer, acknowledging the mistake, apologising to the patient, and informing all involved of the event. Double loop learning would require much more detailed analysis of why this happened in the first place, what the faults and holes in the repeat prescribing system are, what other errors are likely in the current system, how the system can be overhauled to prevent further error and perhaps catastrophe. Double loop learning would look for checks and safety nets within the system and involve other agencies such as pharmacists to improve safety. It requires more effort but produces better results, more effective learning, and in health care is a crucial component of clinical governance.

Implementing change successfully

According to Lewin,[10] effective change occurs when there is dissatisfaction with the current system, the organisation has a shared vision of the future, and there is a safe and acceptable first step. If the momentum generated by these three components is greater than the inertia of the status quo, then there will be change. This model, also referred to as the change equation (see Box 8.1), shows the powers of individuals and teams in not only implementing but also resisting change and can be useful to identify barriers and blocks to change.

Box 8.1 **The change equation.**
Change can occur when A + B + C › D
A = desire for change
B = the vision of how it could be
C = knowledge of the steps needed
D = status quo

Two opposing views of how to bring about change within an organisation have been put forward:

Structure-led approach	Change the structure first, then try to alter behaviour, and finally seek to tackle attitudes.
People-led approach	Involve the staff affected by changing their attitudes first, then their behaviour, and finally the structure.

Structure-led approach

A structure-led approach is very much concerned with formal aspects of change, such as goals, structures, technology, and policies. This will appear logical, planned, and systematic and its benefits will seem obvious to those trying to affect the change. Unfortunately, the approach does not take into account the hurt feelings, resentments, loss of face and status, and anxiety that change can bring about.

People-led approach

The people-led approach is more concerned with looking at the views of individuals regarding the impending change and considering the importance of a feel good factor at work. It is about remembering the importance of motivating factors in an organisational environment (see Chapter 5) and realising that not all are striving for self-actualisation but just trying to attend to basic safety needs such as job security and a work–life balance.

Resistance to organisational change

Change has both positive and negative aspects. On the one hand it implies experiment, innovation, and excitement, while on the other it can also mean discontinuity and the removal of familiar structures and relationships. Despite the positive attributes, change may be resisted because it involves confrontation with the unknown and loss of the familiar.

> *At a practice meeting to discuss the implementation of the new contract, the following discussion was overheard:*
>
> **Dr Angry:** *These targets are just unrealistic, it's ridiculous. How can anyone be expected to reach them? It's not what I trained as a doctor for. It will adversely affect my relationship with my patients.*
>
> **Dr Pragmatic:** *Why don't we just get on and do it – all this time spent moaning about it could be spent valuably, helping us reach those targets. There's no point disagreeing when we voted for this. Personally, I want the money.*
>
> **Dr Been-here-before:** *I remember the last new contract, and what a fiasco that was. We ran a load of stupid clinics that produced no overall patient benefit. I propose to do absolutely nothing and wait and see what mistakes others make.*
>
> **Dr Enthusiastic:** *I'm sorry, but I disagree. We are talking about quality outcomes here and this practice should have been aiming for these targets years ago. As far as I can see it's a win-win; patients get better care and we get richer.*

Bedeian[11] outlined four common causes of resistance to organisational change:

Parochial self-interest

It is human nature to protect a status quo that appears advantageous and offers contentment. Change may threaten our comfort zone and move us away from familiar things that we enjoy. Change may imply loss of power, prestige, approval, status, and security. It may also affect long-standing relationships that have taken time to establish and offer stability and support.

Misunderstanding and lack of trust

Change is much more likely to be resisted if the reasons behind it are not apparent and resistance may therefore be reduced by good communication and transparency behind the changes.

Contradictory assessments

Individuals vary in the way that they view the benefits and costs of change. What can appear exciting to one may be a major threat to another. Individually held values may ultimately determine the types of change that will succeed and those doomed to fail. These contradictions are most apparent when communication is poor and the relevant information is absent. This resistance to change, if listened to and understood, may ultimately lead to a more effective change process.

Low tolerance for change

For some people change implies a loss of the known and familiar and a need to tolerate uncertainty and this can challenge their self-perception and erode confidence. This threat to self-esteem may lead them to resist even obviously beneficial changes. Gaining an understanding of how an individual views this change can help decrease resistance. As Covey[12] says, in order to get your point across 'seek first to understand, then be understood'.

Force-field analysis

Force-field analysis is a technique that can be used to tackle a specific problem in a systematic way with a view to achieving a goal. It is a method of mapping out the forces at work in any situation that are keeping things as they are. Its use helps to diagnose the current situation clearly and to show how it may be changed.

The idea underlying force-field analysis is that, in any apparently stable situation, there is a state of dynamic tension between the forces driving change and those resisting it. This technique sets out these forces diagrammatically, showing their direction and their strength, and then proceeds to show how they can be modified (Figure 8.3). In order to achieve the desired goal, the aim is to reduce or remove the constraining forces. Force-field analysis is useful in formulating action plans following decision making and implementing change effectively.

There are five basic rules to follow in force-field analysis:

Establish workable goals. Need to state goal or desired state in a manner that makes it appear achievable.

Brainstorm methods to achieve goal. List all the restraining forces and the driving forces helping you reach your goal. Highlight the most important forces currently. List all possible actions to eliminate each restraining force and similarly list possible actions to facilitate the driving forces.

Choose the means to achieve goals. Select practical action plans that have high probability of success. Order action plan to move step wise towards the goal. List the steps for each driving force to enhance its potential.

Figure 8.3 **Force-field analysis**

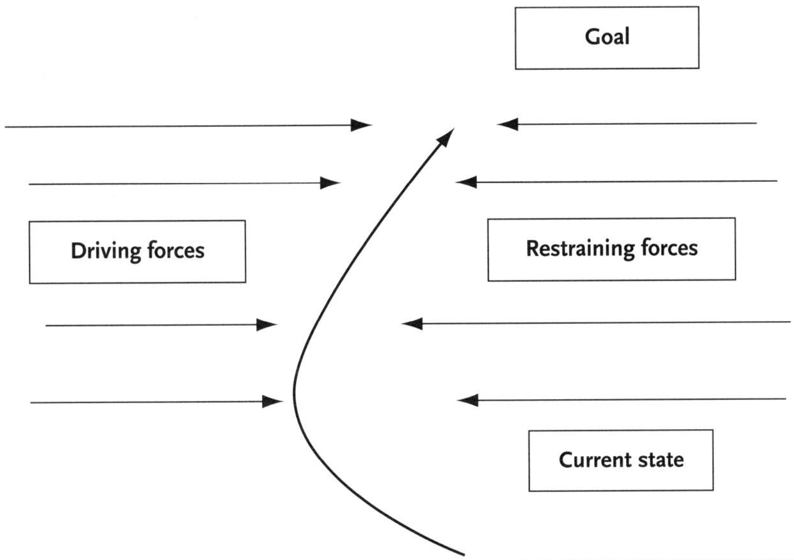

Establish criteria for the effectiveness of plan. What will be the markers of success?

Implementation. Use your chosen plan to achieve the goal.

Try this at home
Think of an example of a change you would like to implement and then summarise it in exact terms. It can be organisational or personal.
- Identify the restraining and driving forces; e.g. personal characteristics, things, individuals involved, etc.
- Identify the forces on each side that appear to be most powerful and give these your attention.
- Look at resisting forces in turn and identify methods of diminishing them.

Skills necessary when leading change
Moss Kanter, one of the leading writers on change, summarises issues that she considers are important in the leadership of change:[8]

Tune into the environment and listen to the workforce, and try to bring into the open the tacit knowledge among the staff. It is necessary to be sensitive towards people's feelings and create individual solutions for individual circumstances, offering alternative flexible arrangements to suit individual needs.

Challenge current wisdom and ask why you've always done things this way. Examine your mental models and paradigms and re-frame ideas, aiming for continuous improvement and quality.

Communicate a compelling aspiration and promote your vision by effective communication and a clear view of the future. You cannot sell change without genuine conviction.

Build coalitions involving those people with the knowledge, resources, and influence to bring about the required change. Although this sounds obvious, it is often one of the most neglected steps. In the early stages identify key allies and change agents who will help ensure success.

Transfer ownership to the working team and let them develop the idea and implement it, although as leader you need to stay involved offering support, coaching, and resources. This approach encourages team ownership and new possibilities and ideas to be explored. Do not, however, simply pile too much responsibility onto team members.

Learn to persevere as the stickiest moments of change are in the middle and it is tempting to launch change and then move onto the next project. Change, once accepted, still does not go smoothly, as forecasts change, the unexpected may well happen, momentum for change slows, and critics emerge during the implementation.

References

1. Handy C. *The Age of Unreason*. London: Arrow Books, 1989.
2. Toffler A. *Future Shock*. London: Pan Books, 1970.
3. Kubler-Ross E. *On Death and Dying*. Toronto: Macmillan, 1969.
4. Handy C. *The Empty Raincoat*. London: Arrow Books, 1994.
5. Harvey-Jones J. *Managing to Survive: a guide to management through the 1990s*. London: Heinemann, 1993.
6. Argyris C, Schön D. *Organisational Learning*. Cambridge, MA: Addison-Wesley, 1978.
7. Senge P. *The Fifth Discipline: the art and practice of the learning organisation*. New York: Doubleday Currency, 1990.
8. Moss Kanter R. *The Enduring Skills of Change Leaders*. Leader to Leader Institute (13). www.pfdf.org/leaderbooks/l2l/summer99/kanter.html, 1999.
9. Mintzberg H, Ahlstrand B, Lampel J. *The Strategy Safari*. New York: Free Press, 1998.
10. Lewin K. *Field Theory in Social Science*. New York: Harper and Row, 1951.
11. Bedeian A. *Organisation Theory and Analysis*. Illinois: Dryden Press, 1980.
12. Covey S. *The Seven Habits of Highly Effective People*. London: Simon and Schuster, 1989.

Chapter 9

In Pursuit of Quality

John Schofield

Each day the Controllers held a conference at which every idea or device for thinking and acting one step ahead of their cunning and resourceful foe was set forth, earnestly discussed and, if found useful, adopted.

HMSO, *The Battle of Britain* (1940)

> **KEY MESSAGES**
> - Listen to what people tell you.
> - Motivate the workers.
> - Always look at things from the customer's point of view.
> - If you can steal a good idea, do!
> - And remember, quality is not just for Christmas!

What's in this chapter

Quality is a term that has been much used and abused in the health service. Despite this, the concept has great virtue and the ideas around quality really are 'people friendly'. Quality is about helping the people you manage in a way that they appreciate while giving them pride and satisfaction in the job they are doing. Motivation, of course, is the key to all of this (see Chapter 5).

In this chapter I cover some theoretical ideas relating to quality and some thoughts on how these might be applied in today's Primary Care environment. I have not gone into details on the 2003 General Medical Services contract, as this deserves (and indeed is) a book on its own.

Theoretical concepts in quality

- The customer
- The team
- The feedback loop
- 'Getting it Right'
- 'Just in Time'

- 'Just for You'
- Enhancement
- Coping with complexity
- Drivers for change

The customer

The ideal quality system is designed to focus on the 'customer' and provide a product or service that more than meets the expectation of the person who is paying the bill. Life gets more complicated in the National Health Service (NHS), as the bill is picked up by the state and ultimately paid for through taxation. Conflict arises, then, when we have to balance the wishes of a given patient at a particular time with the needs of other (potential) patients and the requirements of the government, which in turn is trying to keep health care expenditure within manageable bounds and yet keep the population in a fit and healthy state.

The idea of putting the customer, or patient, at the centre of our organisation may seem obvious, but when one looks around it is astonishing how often you find that systems are set up for the convenience of others. How many hospital outpatient clinics used to book all patients for 2pm when the clinic was due to last all afternoon? Once one has moved away from the concept of the illness belonging to the doctor, to it being in the domain of the patient, then all sorts of possibilities emerge to improve the quality of care. The management of chronic illness, in particular, can be improved by accessing the expert knowledge of the patient. The *BMJ* recently devoted an entire issue to this way of working, in which former Chief Medical Officer, Liam Donaldson, argues the case for the 'expert patient'.[1]

We shall look at ways of focusing on the patient's needs later ('Just for You', page 108).

The team

Traditionally, medicine has been organised in a very hierarchical fashion with the doctor dictating what should be done. There are virtues in knowing where the buck stops, but a quality organisation will also make use of the power of the team to accomplish greater feats than individuals can ever dream of. What we are looking for is clear direction, drive and motivation combined with a process of continual training and retraining, then allowing those who have a job to do to get on with it within their competencies.

From the customer's point of view there is no great virtue in having their blood pressure measured by a stressed doctor when they will happily see a health care assistant or use an automatic machine at home. In many ways demographic changes, new technology, and expectations are driving this process. From a quality perspective, the objective of monitoring a patient's blood pressure can be achieved in a wide variety of ways, ranging from a specialist appointment at £100 a time, to a £50-loan of a sphygmomanometer, which would last many years. Such choices become important issues when a Primary Care Trust (PCT) has to consider how best to spend its budget. In circumstances like these, the power of the team comes into play; a brainstorming session, for instance, will throw up all sorts of innovative ideas. Effective team working is explored in Chapter 4.

The feedback loop

Much of the development of quality theory (and practice) originated in the manufacturing industry. As products became more complex, the notion of an artisan producing a homemade item to sell no longer worked. Things really came to a head when the first complex electrical goods, such as telephones, started to be made. Every component had to work properly or the whole thing was useless. Shewhart[2] was an early contributor to the field with his proposal of a method of continuous improvement, a feedback loop known as the Plan–Do–Study–Act (PDSA) cycle.

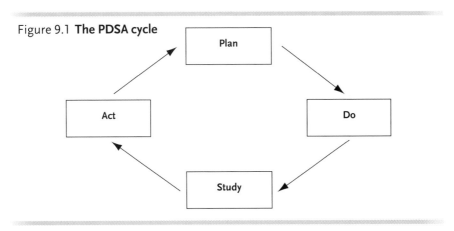

Figure 9.1 **The PDSA cycle**

The PDSA cycle

The seemingly simple idea of actually planning what you were going to do and then looking at the results and making improvements was a revelation. PDSA does mean, as well, that everyone in the team needs to be party to the overall plan and involved with the checking process. There may be ways that this can work in your own organisation.

'Getting it Right'

'Getting it Right' is what *Total Quality Management (TQM)* and *Quality*

Assurance (QA) are all about: one has to constantly review systems and look for ways to improve them. 'Getting it Right' is also concerned with anticipating problems, listening to the workers, and doing something about risks before there is a disaster. An important part of this is for all involved to be 'singing from the same hymn sheet' and looking for the root cause of problems.[3] Entwined in this is the vogue for *significant event analysis* (see Chapter 3, page 32) and *near miss analysis,* both of which were pioneered by the aerospace industry.

The concept of *risk analysis* is also helpful in this field. The idea is to look for potential risks, put in place control measures to cope with them, and then try to quantify any remaining risks.

My personal favourite technique is *Poka–Yoke,*[4] which has two aspects. Firstly, you try to design a product or service so that it can't be used in the wrong way and secondly, even if this should fail, an alarm goes off to warn you. A good example in hospital medicine is the anaesthetic machine that will only allow the gas lines to be connected the correct way. Likewise, in Primary Care, our computerised prescribing programmes make it very difficult to prescribe penicillin to a patient allergic to it.

'Just in Time'

The concept of 'Just in Time' was first developed by the car manufacturer Toyota in response to shortages of available equipment in post-war Japan (well described in Monden's book, *Toyota Production System*; see 'Further reading'). The underlying idea of doing things just as they were required spawned a complex web of interlocking supply chains that could respond very rapidly to changing pressures within the system. Much of our thinking in health care is still stuck with the 19th century tendency to build bigger and grander structures instead of looking for where best services can be delivered to the customer.

In a rapidly changing world with new technologies and new ideas constantly being thrown up, those managing medical care need to develop an open-minded approach. Additionally, the recently acquired easy access to computing power has given us all the ability to look at what we are doing and ask searching questions.

'Just for You'

As patients, what we would all like is a bespoke product that fits our particular needs and wants. 'Just for You' is a developing area in commercial quality circles and has great resonance in health care. Its application in medicine is dependent on the move to a team service approach, the use of near patient technology, the full application of the next generation of IT systems, and the concept of networks.

In theory, it should be possible to develop health care systems that are both responsive to the needs of the patient and able to adapt in appropriate ways to dynamic and changing circumstances. From a management point of view this means focusing on the customer and not being hamstrung by old ideas of how services should be delivered. Modern hospitals are ideal for doing high-tech things well. If you need your hip replaced then that is the place to be. Well before the operation, though, there needs to be a structure in place with procedures, protocols, and care pathways that will quickly and efficiently move the patient through 'the system'. Such 'seamless care' will involve a network of key people and the ability to remotely monitor the patient's progress.

One interesting point about networks is that although there is the expectation that all connections are equal, in fact nodes arise that are vital to the connectability of the whole organisation – these represent the key people that managers need to identify.

Enhancement
By definition – *to raise up.*

It is a central tenet of the quality movement that we will improve every day in small ways and in time will astound the world – the inevitability of the gradual. Quality is an evolutionary process with both positive and negative feedback loops. The bedrock of the process relies on the freedom to be able to talk about both our successes and our failures, without which we will continue to bury (literally in medicine!) our mistakes and will not progress. How we move to a blame avoidance culture I do not know; it seems endemic in human nature. The great guru of health improvement, Donald M Berwick recently wrote: 'So far, I do not find evidence that health care in the United States is becoming safer'.[5] One needs in this process of enhancement to appreciate that everyone has great ideas every day of their life. Invention is not the preserve of the boffin but inbuilt in all of us; all management has to ask is, 'How can we do this better?'

My own experience of work in General Practice, PCTs, and Health Authorities is that the people doing the job are the ones who know best how it works. An apparently straightforward request to work through a flow chart of how the post is dealt with in the morning will generate a host of differing ideas about how best to do it. Old-fashioned technology in the form of a group of people involved with the process and a flip chart is the key to success. Once a system has been agreed on then it is put on a word processor as a procedure and distributed to everyone. The joy of word processing is that it is not set in stone and the procedure can frequently be revisited without any great effort. Audit, done frequently and simply, gives one a feel for how you are progressing and is essential in the feedback loop.

Coping with complexity

Management is about knowing your own limitations. There is a temptation to tie everything down with endlessly more convoluted instructions and try to do everyone else's job yourself. This must be resisted. There are those areas at work that are straightforward and readily controlled and there are those of complete chaos. Between is the zone of complexity, where most of our work is done. By understanding the theoretical basis of complexity one may gain an insight into how best to manage people. (Readers are pointed in the direction of Kieran Sweeney's and Frances Griffiths' book, *Complexity and Health Care*; see 'Further reading').

Drivers for change

Financial. Health care will inevitably consume more of our nation's gross domestic product in the future as people aspire to better health and a longer life of activity and fun. Quality has been identified as a potential vehicle by which these aspirations can be met without bankrupting the country. By doing our work in the NHS better and more consistently, and by using the best evidence available, there is the hope that we may be able to achieve some of the gains seen in the commercial world. Indeed, one only has to look at the inside of a modern PC to wonder not that it occasionally crashes but that it ever works in the first place. This success has been brought about by three aspects of evolutionary theory:

1. Building on what you have.
2. Cross-fertilisation.
3. Extinction and recycling.

What one is looking for is to try and keep the net costs as low as possible by investing sufficiently in system development, training, audit, etc. As the quality of the system improves, the costs come down. (See Figure 9.2.) The dilemma is that the graphs are steadily shifting, so that people accept improvements that are made and are looking for the next thing. Thus, to even stand still one has to be improving the quality of service continually.

Political agendas. Governments find themselves in an impossible position. They have to promise everything to get elected and are immediately blamed when things go wrong. But there is a groundswell of opinion around the world that something has to be done to reduce the disasters that have happened recently in health care. The nightmare scenarios outlined in the Bristol and Shipman Inquires could and should have been avoided. A properly audited quality health system picks up potential problems before they get out of hand.

Figure 9.2 **The cost/quality relationship**

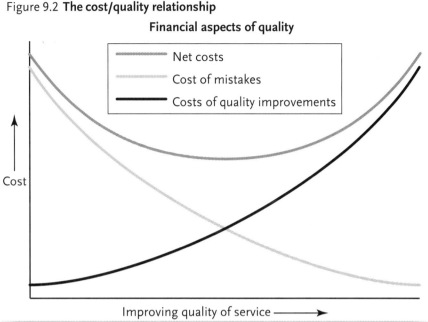

Financial aspects of quality

Litigation. An increasing proportion of what we spend on health goes on compensation claims. By doing things well in the first place and reducing the rate of mistakes the hope is that some of this money can be used in prevention rather than compensating patients for disasters. The NHS has over recent years tried to bring into place systems for making these changes. *A First Class Service: quality in the new NHS*[6] and *The NHS Plan: a plan for investment, a plan for reform*[7] lay out the government's ideas on the way forward. The creation of the National Patient Safety Agency (NPSA)[8] is now leading to some of these changes being implemented.

Technological change. Quality and technology go hand in hand, feeding off one another. As each new invention is brought on stream there has to be an equal if not bigger investment in changing the ways we work, retraining everyone, and, most importantly, thinking very hard about what we are trying to do. The challenge is not with new technology itself but the ability to apply it in people friendly ways.

If you are involved with managing new projects, then there are a few things that are important:
- Involve everyone, the cleaner included, right from the start.
- Aim for small, achievable goals within a short time frame.
- Keep reviewing progress and feed back on how thing are going.

- Try to get your supplier to demonstrate a happy user of the product.
- Focus on what it will mean for the patient (or customer).

Probably the biggest gains from the new IT will be the ability to carry out audit in real time and greater availability of high-quality information leading to increased patient empowerment.

Demographic change. We can't continue to deliver health care as we did. A crunch time is coming when there won't be sufficient young people to look after the old. There are a number of solutions to this dilemma, but one thing we must do is to improve the quality of our systems so that there is less waste, less mistakes, and more flexible systems.

Practical applications

There's nothing like having a go to get an understanding of how you can improve things. First of all, a few musts for any health care organisation.

1. *Folder of procedures*
    Simple, clear procedures are the key to everything. Ideally, they are written by the people doing the job and are reviewed at least yearly. Flow charts can help with clarity of organisation, or a grid with time on one axis and the different people involved on the other works well. Procedures state the obvious to you but maybe not to others.

2. *Folder of protocols and guidelines*
    Doctors have tended to find the idea of these rather threatening, as they – rightly – argue that each patient is an individual. When you analyse cases, however, many aspects are repeated and can be mechanised, with a reduction in stress and the risk of mistakes. One is left with 10–15% of situations needing individual assessment.

3. *A practice/clinic/hospital formulary*
    Again a difficult area, but one that forces people to argue for how they manage particular conditions. A good way of starting is to list all the drugs that clinicians use under the British National Formulary headings and then try to see if there is agreement about reducing the choice. Over a number of years my experience has been that by using a limited list everyone gains.

4. *A duplicate book for messages*
    You can use a large diary but a self-duplicating book works very well. The key point here is that there is an audit trail so that one can always go back to the original message.

5. **A data management policy**

   You have to think about why you are recording data and then you can hopefully make sense of it. We have had an A4 sheet of basic READ codes stuck next to every PC terminal for years. By agreeing to use the same codes throughout a PCT, it is easy to compare results and produce benchmarks.

6. **A routine audit process**

   Quality means continuous feedback. Your PCT may well have an audit and computer group facilitator who will help the practice set up routine and repeatable audits.

7. **A register for recording complaints, near misses, significant events, and thanks**

   It is painful to receive complaints when you are trying to do your best, but they can be used constructively. In my own practice, we keep a log of when patients have been given the wrong drug. This acts as a valuable learning aid to see where mistakes have happened and is a spur to change our procedures (see 'Single and double loop learning', page 98).

8. **Information leaflets, printable from computer**

   One of the features of modern clinical computer systems is the availability of constantly updated information about every conceivable condition at the press of a button. I have two printers set up, one for prescriptions and one to print out the information for patients. They seem pleased.

9. **A supply of 'Patient Care Plans' A5 or A6 size**

   A great breakthrough suggested by a GP registrar. These are designed on A4 and then reduced with the photocopier. The sheet covers lots of routine things to do; e.g. blood tests, urine tests, clinics to attend. I would thoroughly recommend them to you.

10. **A supply of 'Referral Information Forms'**

    Again, a simple sheet with the telephone numbers of the local hospitals and the consultant and specialist that you are referring the patient to.

> *I recently took a sample of our adult patients in the practice and recorded how often they where seeing a health care worker. The results showed that 20% of the patients were using 80% of the resources. Breaking the results down further we found that a particular patient was seen 25 times whilst 14 patients were not seen at all. Is the 25 times a year patient in real need of this frequency of contact or have they some underlying need that has not been addressed? Maybe we should be more concerned about the 14 that*

have not been seen, some of them for more than five years.

If we are trying to provide a good quality service within the constraints of a defined budget and limited manpower, then this type of information offers the opportunity to discuss, with the entire team, whether there are any options available for change or improvement.

Try this at home

- Organisational redesign:
  Ask the team to individually write down what jobs they do on Post-Its and then discuss whether there are any better ways of doing this work.
- Epilepsy audit:
  Plan how you could identify all the epileptic patients in your practice using various search methods.
- Network nodes:
  Write down the names of everyone in the organisation on Post-Its. Put these on a flip chart with lines connecting the people up.
- Flow chart:
  Get the team to devise a flow chart of how hospital letters are managed in the practice and important information recorded and acted on. How could this be done better?
- Borrowing ideas:
  Visit another practice. Steal their good ideas.

References

1. Donaldson L. *Expert patients usher in a new era of opportunity for the NHS.* BMJ 2003; **326**: 1279–1280.
2. Shewhart WA. *Economic Control of Quality of Manufacturing Product.* New York: Van Nostrand, 1931.
3. www.dti.gov.uk/mbp/bpgt/m9ja00001/m9ja0000110.html. (Accessed 1.09.03.)
4. www.qmt.co.uk/courses/quality/poka_yoke.htm. (Accessed 1.09.03.)
5. Berwick D. Errors Today and Errors Tomorrow. *New Eng J Med* 2003; **348**: 2570–2572.
6. Department of Health. *A First Class Service: quality in the new NHS.* London: DOH, 1998.
7. Department of Health. *The NHS Plan: a plan for investment, a plan for reform.* London: DOH, 2000 (www.nhs.uk/nhsplan).
8. National Patient Safety Agency: www.npsa.nhs.uk.
9. NHS – The Improvement Network:
   www.tin.nhs.uk/sys_upl/templates/DblLeft/DblLeft_disp.asp?pgid=1135&tid=75.

Further reading
Journals
Quality and Safety in Health Care. Published by BMJ Journals and the Institute for Healthcare Improvement.

International Journal for Quality on Health Care. Published by Oxford University Press.

Books
Muir JA. *Evidence-based Healthcare: how to make health policy and management decisions.* Edinburgh: Churchill Livingstone, 2001.

Oakland JS. *Total Quality Management.* Oxford: Butterworth Heineman, 1989.

Sweeney K, Griffiths F. *Complexity and Health Care: an introduction.* Abingdon: Radcliffe Medical Press, 2002.

Brooks J, Borgardts I. *Total Quality in General Practice.* Abingdon: Radcliffe Medical Press, 1994.

Nicholson N. *Managing the Human Animal.* London: Texere Publishing, 2000.

Monden Y. *Toyota Production System: an integrated approach to Just-In-Time.* Norcross, GA: EMP Books, 1998.

Chapter 10

Making Meetings Meaningful

David Claridge

Meetings produce minutes and consume hours.

A camel is a horse designed by a committee.

 KEY MESSAGES

Common causes of difficulties in meetings

- Purposes not commonly understood or agreed.
- 'Hidden agendas'.
- Personal egos and beliefs such as 'co-operation' mean 'you do things my way'.
- Poor interpersonal skills, especially in speaking and listening.
- Inappropriate and unquestioned beliefs about how meetings *should* be run.

How to make meetings more effective

- Be clear about the meeting's purpose *and* purposes for each agenda item.
- Use a three-column agenda.
- Select and use meeting 'tools' skilfully.
- Make notes that serve real purposes.
- Agree the precise functions of the chairperson.
- Be aware of and accept personal responsibility for your own behaviour and its effects.

Why do such phrases produce a wry smile of recognition in most of us? Why do meetings seem to take so long to produce so little? Why do even the most democratic of us sometimes yearn to be an absolute dictator? Why do we so often approach meetings with foreboding?

This chapter suggests some common causes of difficulties in meetings. There follow some tried and tested practical proposals for making meetings more effective, proposals which can be adopted by all members together or by an individual acting alone, whether in the role of chairperson or that of an ordinary member.

The common causes of difficulties in meetings

In my experience, most problem meetings exhibit one, or more, of the following characteristics:

- the absence of commonly understood purposes
- our innate humanity (especially those parts we would rather not admit to)
- preconceptions about the 'correct' way to set up and run a meeting.

The absence of commonly understood purposes

The purposes of many meetings can be hard to perceive. Rarely are they discussed openly. In their absence, we deduce, invent, or presume them. Often we compound the problem by assuming that everyone else shares our presumptions. So, even with the best of intentions, we find ourselves talking at cross-purposes. Purposes lie in the responses to questions such as 'Why are we doing this?', 'What are we hoping to achieve?', 'What benefits should result from doing this?' Purposes help us to determine what is relevant and what isn't. They are a beacon for decision making and they are a yardstick for subsequent reviews of achievement.

The problem can be especially acute in regular meetings. There may have been clear purposes initially, but over the months and years, the circumstances will change, some original purposes are no longer relevant and fresh ones arise. Yet the meetings continue in the way they always have done.

A difficulty with thinking about purposes is that it is easy to be general and hard to be specific. Purposes such as 'to improve communications' are, like motherhood and apple pie, an irrefutably 'good thing'. But they fail to illuminate or energise. We need to know communication between whom, about what sort of things, and to what ends.

'Hidden agendas'. The term crops up early in most conversations about meetings and generally in a pejorative sense. They imply secret and sinister motives indifferent to or against our interests. Certainly some people, motivated by ambition for power (say), may seek to deceive and manipulate others towards their own selfish ends. But I find that they are greatly outnumbered by people of good will, willing to co-operate and wanting to do a good job.

The real problem with purposes is that they lie hidden below the surface of the behaviour we see. Suspecting they may be hidden from us, we imagine them hostile. Often, all that is needed is to seek them and make them explicit.

Our innate humanity (especially those parts we would rather not admit to)

Unless we suffer from an acute lack of self-esteem, most of us prefer our own ideas to those of others. We often even prefer our own words to express an idea that someone else has perfectly well explained a few seconds before. There are even some of us who really do love the sound of our own voice. In Peter Shaffer's play *Amadeus*, at the end of the first performance of *Il Seraglio* the Emperor Josef II tells Mozart:

. . . there are simply too many notes, that's all. Just cut a few and it will be perfect.[1]

The same advice applies to most meetings. There are too many words, words that are repetitious, irrelevant, mischievous, or simply a waste of time. But what is the cause of this excess? Let us for a moment reflect on what happens when:

- someone speaks
- s/he is listened to (or not!)
- someone else responds
- the first speaker reacts.

Someone speaks. Naturally, it is in order to convey their thoughts. But is it always that simple? Do we not sometimes speak to impress, pull rank, or intimidate? Do we not sometimes speak to ingratiate ourselves or even to deflect or confuse? Do we always consider the language we use to best help others to listen and understand what we say? Do we blurt something out as soon as the idea comes into our head? Or do we choose the timing by holding back our wonderful proposal to solve the problem until others have really understood what the problem is? As the speaker, we have a vested interest in our ideas being listened to, considered, and used. Is it not then sensible for us to launch them in ways that will assist their survival and success?

To *really listen* to another person, so as to understand their words and their meaning, is hard and demands great concentration. The good manners of remaining silent, looking at the speaker, and appearing to listen are not in themselves sufficient.

Why do we listen to another person? To understand what they have to say, naturally! But when 'listening', are we not sometimes just waiting for the other person to finish so that we can say what we are aching to? Do we not sometimes listen for the flaws in their case so that we point them out and help demolish their idea? Do we not sometimes listen for the differences between our own ideas and theirs in order to better promote ours? Management guru Stephen Covey summed this tendency up succinctly:

We sometimes listen less to understand than to reply.[2]

So what can get in the way of listening?

- Our own thoughts, which of course, are *so* good!
- Prejudice about the speaker and a prior assumption about the worth of what is being said.
- Two or more people talking at once.
- Continuous talk with no space in between contributions for thought.
- The speaker's timing and use of inappropriate language.

Then, *someone responds.* Surprisingly often, there is no overt response to what has just been said. There is no acknowledgement of it and what is next said bears no obvious link with what has just been said.

There are then the pseudo acknowledgements and agreements with which we are all familiar:

'Yes, I agree, only . . .'
   'Yes, but . . .'
      'Instead of that, what about . . .'

What follows the three dots is crucial. It may be that the first two responses do indeed point to a legitimate concern (ideally, but rarely, followed by a proposed solution). But all too often, what follows is a new and quite unrelated idea, that of the second speaker. In this case, the phrases can be translated to:

'I don't agree and I've got a better idea . . .'
   'No, and this is my thought . . .'
      'Here's my alternative . . .'

In the privileged position of coaching small working groups, I have sometimes asked Susan (who has just said 'Yes, I agree, only . . .') to summarise what, in Peter's suggestion, she was agreeing to. It can be a cruel question and humiliating for Susan to have difficulty in answering.

Another familiar response that normally presages an attack is, 'With respect . . .' If you hear 'With the greatest respect . . .' then you know you are in big trouble!

The first speaker may *now react.* S/he may conclude, reasonably enough, that their contribution wasn't listened to and perhaps not even heard. This may lead to:

- a determination to re-state the idea more forcibly and repeatedly if necessary
- a vow to retaliate by ignoring or finding fault with other's contributions
      (both of which add to the wasted word count)
- withdrawal from the contest – 'Why should I bother?'
      (which reduces the word count but defeats the goal of inclusion).

Box 10.1 **What is happening at this practice meeting?**

Charles: *Can we now turn to the staff appraisal scheme. We agreed at the last meeting that the present system doesn't really work and has become a bit of a joke. It needs revising and Mary offered to put up an 'Aunt Sally' to help us start our discussion at this meeting.*

Mary: *Which I did. Did everyone get a copy? Did you find time to read it?*

(A few murmurs of 'Yes')

John: *I got it but haven't got round to reading it, I'm afraid. Last week was horrendous, what with having to give evidence in that court case. Sorry.*

Anne: *What court case was that? You must tell me about it because I may find myself in a similar position.*

Charles: *Well, no matter. I suggest we go round the table to hear everyone's first thoughts. Who'll start?*

(Silence for 10 seconds)

Alan: *You might remember that I wasn't at the last meeting. I don't know what this is about.*

Mary: *Shall I start since I've already done a bit of thinking.*

Sue: *Oh no! We know your ideas already. We should hear everyone else's.*

Mary: *Fine, so who's first?*

John: *I'll start then. Whatever system we have, it should be to do with personal development and not influence what we pay people.*

Anne: *For heaven's sake, how do you recognise good or bad performance if it isn't reflected on the pay packet in some way.*

Mary: *Perhaps with a kind word and a 'thank you', which I think we are all pretty bad at doing.*

Sue: *Kind words don't pay grocery bills.*

Alan: *Please, what is all this about?*

Peter: *Will it help us to get rid of that dead wood in reception?*

Charles: *I think we should approach it more positively than that.*

Sue: *I assume that as partners, we won't be directly involved in it. I don't have the time for yet more administration.*

Mary: *Oh, but I think we should. It's all 360 degree appraisal nowadays you know.*

Peter: *What's that then?*

Sue: *Look, I'm only half-time and yet I regularly turn in between 30 and 35 hours per week. I came into medicine to treat patients, not fill forms.*

Alan: *Since when has there been a standard working week for doctors?*

Charles: *Can we get back to the point please?*

Preconceptions about the 'correct' way to set up and run meetings

I am repeatedly amazed at meeting agendas that start:

1. *Apologies for absence*
2. *Minutes of the last meeting*
3. *Matters arising*
   a)
   b)
   c)

and end with that notorious Pandora's box:

8. *Any other business*

simply because someone believes that this is how meetings 'ought' to be run, regardless of the nature of the meeting.

There are occasions, of course, when formality is necessary; for example, meetings that have to meet statutory requirements. Similarly, highly detailed minutes of who said what might be required for historical or legal reasons. But the majority of meetings held in Primary Care are not of that nature. Ritual and tradition make us comfortable. They save us from thinking. But to be effective, meetings need much thought.

Other common preconceptions, perhaps worth re-assessing, are that:

- all meetings must have a chairperson
- the chairperson should be the most senior person present
- minutes will be taken by an appointed person, often the most junior who is least able to understand the issues under discussion
- arcane language, never used in other circumstances, is acceptable... 'Through the chair, I would like to move a point of order'
- voting is a good way of reaching decisions. It may well force a decision, but it will not achieve consensus or commitment.

How to make meetings more effective

The following suggestions are made with meetings of four or more people in mind. Most of them are relevant to smaller meetings too, even meetings between just two people. The principles also apply to video-link or other electronic meetings. Like all tools and techniques, one needs to become familiar with them and then select and use them with skill to suit the circumstances.

They are offered under five headings:

1. Overall purposes and planning of meetings.
2. The three-column agenda.

3. Other useful procedures and techniques.

4. Meeting notes/minutes.

5. The role of the chairperson.

More fundamental than such 'tools' however is an awareness of one's own values and concomitant behaviour, coupled with a sensitivity to the effects of our behaviour on others and on the progress of the matter in hand. Each of us is accountable for these and, therefore, we hold the seeds of change in our own hands.

1.   Overall purposes and planning of meetings

Meetings are expensive in terms of time. So they need to be well-planned. There should be real clarity about the purposes the meeting will serve: what is it for? what benefits should it bring? The answers need to be specific if they are to produce an 'a-ha' reaction from those who will be involved:

> A-ha – these are really useful things to do. I can see some very tangible benefits and I can see how a meeting will help achieve them.

Beware statements that elicit a 'So, what's new?' reaction. Good purposes energise and motivate people.

In the light of these purposes, who should attend? Does everyone need to be present at every meeting? ... for the whole of each meeting? ... is a varying composition viable? For regular meetings, how often should they be and roughly for how long?

Such thinking is better for being discussed and agreed by all involved and perhaps other stakeholders too.

Remembering that purposes can change over time, review them periodically, say every six or 12 months.

> Some years ago, I was promoted and so became a member of a monthly meeting of about a dozen people, most of whom had been attending the meetings for far longer than I. They all hated the meetings and frequently complained about them to each other. 'It's a complete waste of time' was the common view. I soon came to be of the same opinion and even entered into the 'Ain't it awful' chats.
>
> The only person apparently not of this view was the director in charge and who, of course, was always the chairman. He dominated the meetings and ran them very formally, the way he always had done. The meetings consisted mainly of a series of one-to-one conversations between the director and each departmental head in turn, with the others totally

disinterested because experience had taught them that their contributions were not welcomed. The odd group discussion centred very much on the chairman and on what he wanted to say.

About 12 months after I joined the meeting, another newcomer started coming. She started to display the same symptoms as me: bewilderment followed by increasing frustration. But at her third meeting she chose her moment and asked the chairman directly, 'As you know Mr Chairman, I've only just started attending these meetings and I'm finding it difficult to know how best to prepare and contribute to them. Could you please help me? What are the purposes of these meetings and what should we be getting out of them?'

There was complete silence. Everyone was listening now. The chairman, flattered by being asked for help, and with some magnanimity, started to respond to the question. But he soon got into difficulty and waffled dreadfully because he had never really thought about it himself until then.

But, *one of the senior people said, 'Well, I always thought they were . . .' 'Oh no, I thought the point was to . . .' said another. And then another spoke, and another. Some suggested what the benefits could be. For the first time in several years, this senior group of managers started thinking and discussing why they met for two hours every month and what benefits they wanted to get out of it. It wasn't easy and it dragged on for another two or three meetings. But thereafter, meetings were shorter, more focused, more productive, and no longer considered a waste of time. In fact, over time, they became one of the cornerstones of managing that division.*

And all because the most junior member asked the right question at the right time, in the right way.

2.   The three-column agenda

All meetings should have an agenda. Sometimes, this may be compiled and distributed in advance. Other times, it can be produced at the start of the meeting (and recorded on a flip chart for all to see). Even if produced in advance, the agenda should be confirmed at the start of the meeting, with opportunities to add or delete items, change the order, or amend the timings. Agreed changes should be noted on a flip chart.

In short, the first item on every agenda should read, 'Confirm/amend the agenda for this meeting'.

Conventionally, agenda items are one- or two-word headings. If the discussion is to be focused and relevant, we need to know the purposes of each item.

This is what the three-column agenda is for:

Item	Purposes and Outcome	Time
1.		
2.		
3.		
4.		

Item. This is the familiar heading or topic title. It may also indicate the person who has raised the item or who has the responsibility for following it through and any other references; for example, notes of previously circulated papers.

Purposes and Outcome. These consist of phrases or sentences that answer the following questions:
• Purposes: Why are we addressing this item at this meeting? What benefits will result?
• Outcome: What is the nature of the outcome we want to achieve by the end of this item? For example, an exploration of everyone's views, the terms of reference for a project, a decision on future action.

Difficulty in responding to such questions suggests a lack of clarity in the mind of the person proposing that item. It prompts the question whether any time should be spent at the meeting on that topic without further thought.

Time. This column is for the best estimate of the time needed to deal with the agenda item. It forms the basis of a timetable against which to pace the meeting and make adjustments as necessary.

Here are some other suggestions for improving agendas.

'Any other business'. Never leave such an item lurking at the end of the agenda. It may be an unexploded bomb. Instead, ask people to declare 'any other business' items at the outset. Also, require purposes and outcomes to be stated together with a time estimate. If accepted and feasible in the time available, plan them into the agenda. Treat similarly any fresh topics that arise during the course of the meeting. Don't be side-tracked into dealing with them there and then; instead, 'park' them on a flip chart for attention later.

Meeting review. This should always be the final agenda item, even if only five or ten minutes can be spared. Useful questions to ask here are:

What was successful about the way this meeting went? What caused these and how can we make sure that they are repeated in future?

What wasted time or made for other difficulties and how can we avoid similar things next time?

Even if such reviews are not the group norm, any individual can benefit from a review of this kind.

3.   Other useful procedures and techniques

Make use of a flip chart. Everyone is familiar with using a personal note pad to record important information or agreements reached. A flip chart is simply a group note pad that is visible to all. Subsequently typed, it can become the meeting notes (see below). Remember to tear a completed sheet off the pad and attach it to the wall so that it remains visible rather that flip it over and hide it.

Create time to think. A curious phenomenon becomes apparent during most meetings, the assumption that someone must be talking all the time. No sooner does one finish then another starts – and that's without the interruptions! There is wall-to-wall talking and no time to think. In my experience, a person can talk, listen, or think. No one can do two of these simultaneously, not if they are to be done well.

And thinking is best done in silence.

So, when there is a need to think seriously, create some time for it. Propose a two- or three-minute silence, for each to then come up with some considered responses or suggestions. Note that this is not the same thing as a break for people to visit the loo or grab a coffee. It is a group of people together, in silence, reflecting on some common issue. Subsequent contributions are invariably higher in quality and generally more succinct.

Go round the table. Hear everyone's thoughts or proposals in turn, without discussion, and capture them on the flip chart. Only then discuss them. In some ways, this is similar to 'brainstorming', but being ordered, especially if preceded by a pause to reflect, it tends to produce better material.

Summarise frequently. This is especially useful when starting to feel bogged down.

Remember, anyone can propose such procedures at any time; it is not solely the chairperson's prerogative to do so.

4.   Meeting notes or minutes

Once again, the critical question is: 'What is the purpose of the notes?'

- If they are to remind people who attended the meeting of things agreed to be done, by whom and by when, the notes can be terse and confined to just these points. If a flip chart has been used to record these during the meeting, a typed transcript of the chart will often suffice.

- If the notes are to inform others who were not at the meeting, then they will probably need to be fuller; the question then arises of how much detail is necessary.
- If a record has to be kept for statutory purposes, the notes will probably need to be very full and perhaps in a prescribed format . . . proper minutes, in fact.

There is rarely a need for notes of Hansard quality.

5. The role of the chairperson

Firstly consider, is there a role for one? Certainly the more personally competent the members and if they adopt effective behaviours and procedures, the less need there is for a chairperson, at least in a 'controlling' capacity.

None the less, I generally find that a chairperson can contribute greatly to a meeting's success. In any meeting, there are two things to be managed or facilitated:

1. The content, in the form of the agenda items.
2. The process of the human interactions in addressing them.

In respect of the content, the ideal chairperson is impartial and balanced with a facility for drawing things together and summarising. Any person who has a high personal stake in the outcome is unlikely to be a good chairperson, at least in respect of that item. The chairperson's prime responsibility must be to facilitate the process of the meeting – high competence in inter-personal and facilitation skills is called for. The most senior person or the technically most able may, or may not, possess these skills.

Putting it into practice

If you are an ordinary member of a meeting, there are all sorts of things you can do that are in no way dependent upon your status in the meeting.

- In the matter of your personal behaviour in communicating, listening, and responding to others, you clearly have total autonomy. This is your responsibility and you are accountable for what you do and what you fail to do. But that is not all. If you observe a problem in the group and you know something that may help, you can offer your observation openly to the whole group or to the chairperson and suggest a remedy. For example: 'I'm losing track of where this discussion is going. I suggest we go back and remind ourselves what we're trying to achieve' or 'Can someone summarise where we are, because I've lost track?'

- When proposing agenda items of your own, also make explicit the purposes and benefits as you see them, the hoped for outcomes at that meeting, and the time estimate.
- If you are unclear about the purposes of a meeting or a particular agenda item, ask. An approach along the lines of, 'It would help me to know . . . Can you please explain?' is probably going to be more fruitful than an aggressive, 'Why are we doing this?'
- When listening to others, listen for points of agreement, build upon them, and encourage them towards decision and action. Cultivate the mind set of saying 'Yes, and . . .' rather than 'Yes, but . . .'. Look not simply for agreement with your own views but also agreement between others, which may be concealed in different words. Look for and point out the potential for synthesis. Propose ways to do this.
- When highlighting a problem, try also to offer a proposal that will alleviate it.
- Keep an eye on the clock and draw attention to it if the meeting is running late. Perhaps the agenda needs to be re-planned.
- Propose or support procedures and techniques suggested in this chapter, if you believe they may help.
- Act as a monitor on other people's non-listening and, consequently, risk of ideas being lost. This is often easier if it is someone else's idea that is being submerged. 'I think that Anne had a suggestion about this a few minutes ago, but I'm not sure I heard it properly.' This has the gracious secondary effect of leaving the credit with Anne.

If you are the chairperson, then you can do even more because you have added authority.

- You can insist on a three-column agenda and refuse to accept agenda items that have not been fully thought through.
- You can refuse a new item proposed near the end of the meeting and defer it to another occasion.
- You can cut down irrelevancies by reminding the authors that they don't seem to help towards the current purposes.
- You can propose techniques and procedures with far more clout than can ordinary group members.
- You can watch out for the quieter, more retiring members who are inclined to be trampled underfoot and give them your support and protection.
- Above all, maintain your awareness of the total situation and keep a certain distance from the detail of the discussion. You need to be seen as impartial. If you can't be, propose that a colleague take over the chair, perhaps just for that agenda item.

In conclusion...

Unlike *Il Seraglio*, at a meeting, the fewer the words, the better. The greater the amount of thought and the more ordered the proceedings, the more effective it will be. It may then be possible to feel:

Great! I've got a day full of meetings. We'll be able to get all manner of things sorted out now.

References

1. Shaffer P. *Amadeus*. New York: Perennial, 2001.
2. Covey SR. *The Seven Habits of Highly Effective People*. London: Simon and Schuster, 1992.

Chapter 11

Working in Organisations

Jan Pearcey

 KEY MESSAGES

Successful organisations (small or large) have:

- The ability to respond to the rapidly changing environment and demands from within and outside of the organisation.
- A clear understanding by all members of the organisation of the business, vision, and values of the organisation.
- Clarity about what the 'must do' activities are, who performs them, and how they relate to one another.
- A range of systems that help the organisation run smoothly.
- An appraisal and personal development planning process for all staff.
- An organisational culture that ensures organisational objectives are met.
- Good communication and information systems.

This chapter provides a brief overview of what it is to work in an organisation and how organisations work. Topics covered include organisational structure, function, roles, systems, culture, management, communication, and information. This chapter's content is by no means comprehensive, nor does it provide a foolproof recipe for effectiveness, but hopefully, what follows will give the reader some insight into the workings of their own organisation.

Organisational structures

For the purposes of this chapter *organisational structure* describes how an organisation divides its work into specific activities and then co-ordinates them in order to achieve its objectives. There are many examples of different types of organisational structures propounded by theorists such as Henry Mintzberg[1] and Charles Handy.[2] The important thing to remember is that whatever the structure, it must be able to deliver the business of the organisation. No one particular organisational model or structure may give the desired results. An effective organisation ideally needs to have open and flexible styles of management to maximise its ability to be adaptable in response to the constantly changing environment of the business world and, in our case, Primary Care and the National Health Service.

Structural models

Table 11.1 summarises four of the many models of organisational structures to be found in popular management literature.

Table 11.1 **Structural models of organisations.**

Structure	Description	Advantages	Disadvantages
Matrix	Projects are the main way of working, with an expert holding responsibility for a specific piece of work.	Easier to keep an overview of the work of the organisation, as a single individual holds responsibility for each project.	Can create a lot of work requiring extra support staff.
Bureaucratic	Relies upon the predictable behaviour of employees. Responsibility is devolved throughout a generally hierarchical structure.	Can work well in large organisations. Rules and procedures ensure fair treatment of employees.	Lack of flexibility to cope with crisis. Rules and regulations rather than creativity and individual judgement.
Entrepreneurial	Decisions and strategy lay with the Senior Partner, Chief Executive. Business style is aggressive and innovative. The leader can be autocratic or charismatic.	Will be able to take advantage of opportunities to expand and is often more flexible.	The leader has the future of the organisation in his/her hands and may have difficulty delegating.
Independent	Example: Barrister, GP. The lead professional is the main decision maker, with organisational support, if any, in the background.	Only for the lead professional autocratic, top down decision making.	Lack of employee involvement in decision making leading to reduced commitment, creativity, self-direction, and initiative.

Creating organisational structures that work

The first thing to consider in creating an organisational structure that works is the issue of common aims of the organisation. Covey[3] states that one of the chronic problems in organisations is that there is 'no shared vision and values: either the organisation has no mission statement or there is no deep understanding of and commitment to the mission at all levels of the organisation'. An organisation needs to be able to give a clear message to its employees about what its objectives are. This gives direction to individuals, teams, and the organisation as a whole through a message of consistency and coherence. To get commitment, staff need to be involved in the agreement of the vision, values, and objectives of the organisation. This helps to ensure that things happen in the right way, at the right time, and for the right reasons.

Functions

In attempting to create an effective organisational structure it is important to remember that, in an ideal world, form follows function. Early identification of the functions of the organisation can create a good basis for clarifying the roles required to deliver those functions and where they sit in the organisational structure. A planned change management programme may even be required. (The management of change is more fully explored in Chapter 8.)

Let's look at some of the functions of organisations. Table 11.2, based on the work of Henri Fayol,[4] lays out groups of organisational functions mapped onto Primary Care. The list is not exhaustive and you may be able to think of others.

Key components of the organisational structure

Once organisational functions have been identified the next step is to create a structure that allows functions to be carried out in a manner that meets organisational objectives. This, if you like, is creating the skeleton upon which the functions hang.

Chapter 1 has already touched upon the work of Henry Mintzberg, particularly his ground breaking work on organisational design.[1] Mintzberg, you may recall (Figure 1.1, Chapter 1), defined five components of any organisation:

1. *Strategic Apex* – this would be the senior management team or practice partners with overall responsibility for all aspects of the organisation.
2. *Middle Line* – could be the business/practice manager acting as 'chain of command' link between the operating core and the Strategic Apex.
3. *Operating Core* – those who perform the mainstay activities of the organisation, such as the clinical patient services, practice management.
4. *Administrative Support* – closely attached to the operating core and supporting and co-ordinating operating core activity.

Table 11.2 **Organisational functions.**

Function	Example
Technical/clinical	Clinical services offered, specialist services, prescribing, management of the clinical areas, clinical IT systems, service commissioning, health needs assessment
Leadership	Clinical services, innovation, project management, strategy and planning
Commercial	Stock control, marketing the organisation, relationship building with other providers, annual reports and practice development plans, newsletters, user/patient panel
Financial	Business accounting, prescribing activity, salaries and wages, taxation, pensions, insurance, service budgets, resource negotiation
Security and risk	Premises, Caldicott, health and safety, infection control, education and training, record keeping and storage, complaints management, audit
Managerial	Business management, human resource management, links with the Primary Care Trust, links with health and social care providers, Information Management, contractual requirements, practice development, induction training, disciplinary, performance review
Administrative	General administrative and clerical functions, management of information
Communication and information	IT systems, practice meetings, patient information, user groups

5. *Technostructure* – technical support, whether regulatory or operational; e.g. human resources, IT department.

The relative importance of these components and the relationships between them vary depending on the type of organisation, which in turn depends on the organisation's purpose.

Try this at home

Review the core business of your organisation?
- What is the structure of your organisation at present – matrix, bureaucracy, entrepreneurial, independent, a combination?
- Does it support the business of the organisation? If not, why not?
- What are the relationships in your organisation between Mintzberg's structural components: the Strategic Apex, the Middle Line, the Operating Core, Administration, and the Technostructure.

So how does this fit together?

In attempting to create an organisational structure that works, the functions and structural components need to be able to respond flexibly to the challenges of day-to-day business.

Gareth Morgan[5] describes the concept of contingency theory based on the research findings of Burns and Stalker. Contingency theory is based on the premise that in order to develop an organisational structure that works, the environment must be considered.

- Organisations are open systems of working that need careful management to satisfy and balance the internal needs of the organisation and adapt to environmental circumstances.
- There is no one best way of organising. The appropriate form depends of the type of task or environment with which one is dealing.
- Management must be concerned, above all else, with achieving alignments and good fits.
- Different approaches to management may be necessary to perform different tasks in the same organisation.
- Different types of organisations are needed in different types of environments.

Just one more model – the Learning Organisation

Whatever the structure of the organisation its effectiveness can be enhanced through what Senge[6] describes as the 'Learning Organisation' – an environment where people think about how everything relates to everything else, where individuals are encouraged to commit to life-long learning, where there is a shared vision, and where team learning is core to creating an effective organisation.

Senge suggests that an effective organisation is one that is:

- continually expanding people's capacity to create the results they desire
- nurturing new patterns of thinking
- establishing collaboration
- continually discovering how to learn together.

So what will help make your structure work?

There are a number of things that can be done to help an organisation to function effectively whatever its structure:

- *Roles* – that ensure that functions are carried out.
- *Systems* – communication, information, remuneration, education, training and development, recruitment and selection, job design.
- The *culture* of the organisation – how staff work together, interpersonal relationships, values and beliefs, team working.
- *Management and leadership* – where these roles sit in the organisation, managing upwards, downwards, and sideways.
- *Communication* – types and benefits.

Roles

The next step in creating an effective organisational structure is to look at roles and responsibilities that will help the organisation to deliver its functions and meet its objectives.

A key part of this is the creation of roles with job descriptions capturing the functions that deliver the business of the organisation. An organisation can create its own job descriptions, but it is worth contacting the Human Resources department of other, similar organisations who may have specimen job descriptions that can be amended. This saves time and helps ensure that the job descriptions have been evaluated giving an appropriate grade or salary. In creating job descriptions from scratch it is worth using a competency model that will help to make the job description relevant, resulting in a person specification that facilitates the recruitment of an appropriately qualified person. Dorothy Del Bueno[7] describes three skill domains for competence in organisations, which may aid this process:

1. *Technical competency*, which includes knowledge, cognitive skills, technical understanding, psychomotor skills.
2. *Critical thinking competencies*, which include problem solving, time management, priority setting, planning, creativity, co-ordination.
3. *Interpersonal competencies*, which include communication skills, conflict management, facilitation, team skills, collaboration.

Each role will have a different range of competencies within each of the domains.

Job descriptions, person specifications, and recruitment are discussed in detail in Chapter 2.

Try this at home

Quickly review the roles undertaken by personnel in your team or organisation.
- Do existing job descriptions bear any resemblance to what the job holder actually does?
- Are people's roles and responsibilities clear to everyone in the organisation?

Systems

Organisations need a range of suitable systems that help the organisation run smoothly. Most organisations will require the following:

Communication. This may include one-to-one sessions, team and staff meetings, and things like 'good idea' boxes. To increase effectiveness it is important that the communication systems in any organisation are built around the organ-isation's business, vision, and values. Good communication systems can ensure that information is fed throughout the organisation in a consistent manner.

Information. The sharing of organisational objectives, work streams, new proj-ects, protocols and guidelines, and social events must occur through an effective information system. This will give consistent messages about performance, standards and quality, and the commitment of the organisation to keeping people informed.

Remuneration. Pay, conditions, responsibility, opportunity, position, and promo-tion. Effective reward systems include monetary and psychological incentives.

Education, training, and development. Ideally, the organisation will encourage and support self-directed learning in staff. Organisational support and guidance gives individuals and teams a message of commitment to their development and can result in individual learning being passed on to others. Education, training, and development is also a proven staff retention strategy.

Recruitment and selection. Effective organisations and managers select and re-cruit people by matching candidates' skills, abilities, attitudes, and interests with the needs of the job. This is in the best interests of the organisation and the candidate.

Job design. Jobs should be designed to capture the needs of the organisation, its business, vision, and values, as well as the interests and skills, experience, and knowledge of potential candidates. There needs to be clarity about the resources available to do the job and the level of authority or degree of autonomy invested in the role.

Organisational culture – setting the tone

Organisations are made up of the people and each individual will bring their own life experiences, values, beliefs, and problems. The culture of the organisa-tion can also be a reflection of the environment in which the organisation exists, the buildings, ethnic diversity, organisational history, and memory. It is impor-tant that the organisation has a set of values, behavioural and business, that relate to the vision and objectives of the organisation. This helps individuals and teams understand what the standards for behaviour are and also gives the outside world the message about how well the organisation works. As men-tioned at the beginning of the chapter, it is important to ensure that staff contribute to the selection and agreement of these values so that there is owner-ship and consensus about what sets the tone for the organisation's collaborative atmosphere. A healthy organisation culture can also be perpetuated through an effective and meaningful appraisal system (see Chapter 3).

Behavioural values *might include:*	Business values *might include:*
• open and honest communication	• quality
• mutual respect and support	• team working
• listening	• financial probity
• giving feedback	• collaboration/partnership

Healthy interpersonal relationships are maintained if the organisation works within a context of agreed behavioural values and gives consistent and visible support. Developing healthy interpersonal relationships (both internal and external) requires time, effort, and sign-up from all members of the organisation. In reality, this can be difficult to attain – and managers must be seen to 'walk the talk'.

Management and leadership

Management and leadership are terms that are frequently used interchangeably (see Chapter 1 page 4). For the purpose of this chapter, management is that which deals with structures, systems, and processes that help ensure that the organisation meets its objectives. The management style within an organisation can be either *participative*, creating an environment for creativity, innovation, and autonomy, or *autocratic*, leading to dependency, stifling both creativity and the capability for independent problem solving.

Managers have three main areas of responsibility in organisations: *finance*, *personnel*, and *quality*. The structure of the organisation may dictate where managerial and leadership roles sit and what levels of authority these roles have. While leadership roles can be found anywhere in an organisation and are often situational, managerial roles are usually positional within the organisational structure and can be the glue that holds the organisation together. Managers are the link between the senior management team and the operational elements of the organisation and direct and monitor much of the function of the organisation.

Any manager, depending on their position in the organisation, will have a range of responsibilities that entail the development of relationships. These may be:
• upwards with the strategic management team, partners, and external organisations that may performance manage them
• peer relationships with other managers in the organisation
• relationships with staff who may report to them or who they work with on a regular basis.

These relationships are key, particularly when managing the delegation of work.

And delegation raises the issues of responsibility and authority and decision making in the organisation.

Responsibility and authority

> At a recent PCT meeting, Mary has been asked to find out what the uptake of pneumococcal vaccination is within the locality. This, to her, seems an enormous and time-consuming piece of work, she's not sure what will be done with the results, and anyway she has her emails to answer. The audit is put off, Mary keeps quiet in the next meeting, and the next spring arrives. Nobody appears to have noticed.

An understanding of what is meant by responsibility and authority within any organisation can increase effectiveness and the chances of a successful outcome. Managers will often delegate new responsibilities to staff, but during the process of delegation and acceptance of the responsibility three things are often not made clear:

1. What taking responsibility really means.
2. What the level of authority is in relation to the carrying out of the new responsibility.
3. What outcomes might be expected.

It is important when delegating work to be very clear about what is expected of the individual and what their level of authority is in relation to the piece of work. Are they being asked to just gather early information about what form the audit might take with recommendations for proceeding, or are they being asked to manage the whole process from beginning to end without checking back with anyone in the organisation?

If the person delegating is not clear about what is required and the person accepting the responsibility does not ask then it is highly likely that the piece of work will either be delayed, may never happen or be completed, or go completely off track leading to an unexpected outcome.

Decision making. An organisation with a structure that has an open and clear process for decision making is more likely to be effective than one where decisions happen in an ad hoc manner or where the authority to make decisions is invested in a few individuals at the top of the organisation. In a bureaucratic or independent structure the latter is often the case. Staff can become demotivated with the creation of a 'them and us' culture, which can result in resentment at decisions made without consultation. Ultimately, staff will no longer think for themselves and will become dependent on the decision makers or will leave to find an organisation where their opinion counts and is respected. Gaining consensus is difficult in any organisation and it requires people to be able to agree to disagree in an environment where the process for decision making is clear.

> **Try this at home**
> Reflect on the main management style in your organisation.
> - Is it autocratic, participative, charismatic, democratic?
> - Do managers 'talk' participation but 'walk' something else?
> - What might the impact of this be on organisational effectiveness?

Communication

Covey[3] suggests that communication is a 'prerequisite to problem-solving and one of the most fundamental skills in life'. Communication comes down at all levels to how much trust and acceptance there is between individuals and teams. Social, political, professional, cultural, and environmental issues affect the way in which messages are given and received and can cloud what may have started out as a simple piece of two-way communication.

Hersey et al[8] describe five internal organisational communication systems:

1. *Downwards.* The most common form of communication flowing from the manager to the follower. Often written and related to task commands, changes in policies or procedures, performance feedback.
2. *Upwards.* From a subordinate to a manager and can be verbal, non-verbal, or written.
3. *Horizontal.* With peers and less formal, and often involves problem solving.
4. *Grapevine.* Found in all organisations and often forgotten, but can be the most powerful, particularly where there is secrecy, poor communication by management, and autocratic leadership behaviours. Information shared through this route can be between 70–90% accurate.
5. *Networks.* Denotes another informal communication system and consists of regular interactions between groups and individuals and can often be the link between other communication systems.

> **Try this at home**
> Find an example of when some information was communicated well to staff and an example of when some information was communicated badly.
> - What types of internal communication systems predominate in your organisation?
> - What was different about the communication that made it go well on one occasion and badly on another?

Managing information

Organisations, regardless of size, need to have information systems that ensure that all managers and their staff have an accurate and balanced picture of what is happening inside the organisation. As we have just seen, communication happens in many ways and information can get distorted as it passes from individual to individual. There are a number of ways that information can be disseminated throughout organisations and it is important to remember that individuals have preferred ways of absorbing information:

- *Staff briefing*. This can be part of regular team or staff meetings. The information to be given, however, must be agreed, documented, and given in an unbiased manner.
- *Newsletters/bulletins*. Can be a written version of the staff briefing, a staff-led publication, or a combination of the two. Bulletins can also be used for rapid dissemination of important information.
- *Communal/group emails*. Can be used for disseminating important information quickly if all staff have access to IT.
- *Notice boards*. Can also be used to display a broad range of information, including important or urgent bulletins, training, and social events.

The key in all information flows is consistency in terms of the messages being given and to whom they are sent. Also, messages should always be sent in a timely manner. Inconsistency and poor timing can be seen as divisive and can cause conflict. Other more specific issues to be considered are:

Record keeping and storage

Keeping accurate and contemporaneous records has a number of advantages:

- It is easier to follow something up if records, whether written or electronic, are kept in order, up to date, and in safe and organised storage. Filing systems should be aligned and easily searchable.
- Certain types of information have to be kept for a minimum number of years in order to satisfy statutory requirements.
- Records and other forms of information may be required as part of an investigation following any complaints.
- Data protection, Caldicott Guardian, and Freedom of Information principles must be applied.

IT and clinical systems

Keeping and recording information is subject to the same conditions as written record keeping. The key differences are:

- All users of the IT or clinical system need to be inputting information in the same way using the same READ codes. The use of templates and protocols can aid consistency and support audit activity.

- In order to satisfy statutory requirements, back-up systems need to be in place in case of any systems failure, to ensure that all information that needs to be kept for a given period can be retrieved if necessary.

Try this at home

Imagine there has been serious complaint from a member of the public about an episode of clinical care received locally?

- Was any record kept of the incident and where would this information be stored?
- Who would have access to this information on request?
- What might happen if the incident has not been recorded in a timely manner?
- What might happen if the information stored is incomplete?
- Who should have overall responsibility for record keeping and information management in the organisation?

References

1. Mintzberg H. *Structure in Fives: designing effective organisations.* Harlow: Prentice Hall, 1992.
2. Handy C. *Understanding Organisations.* London: Penguin, 1993.
3. Covey S. *Principle Centred Leadership.* London: Simon and Schuster Ltd, 1999.
4. Fayol H. *General and Industrial Administration.* London: Pitman and Sons, 1949.
5. Morgan G. *Images of Organisations.* California: Sage Publications, 1997.
6. Senge P. *The Fifth Discipline.* New York: Doubleday, 2000.
7. Del Bueno D, Griffin LR, Burke SM, Foley MA. The clinical teacher: a critical link in competence development. *Journal of Nursing Staff Development* 1990; **6**: 135–138.
8. Hersey P, Blanchard KH, Johnson D. *The Management of Organisational Behaviour.* Harlow: Prentice Hall, 2000.

Chapter 12

Personal Effectiveness

Jill Edwards

 ### KEY MESSAGES

- Before you manage others, understand yourself.
- Celebrate your strengths and acknowledge your weaknesses.
- Manage your emotions.
- Find a job in which you can experience 'flow'.
- Work isn't everything.

This chapter discusses the importance of understanding and managing ourselves before we can begin to manage others effectively. Understanding ourselves will also help us to make more 'best-fit' career choices and achieve that difficult balance between work and life.

Understanding ourselves

Before you can even begin to manage others you need to manage yourself. The key to self-management is understanding our personality and our emotions.

> *Anyone can become angry – that is easy. But to be angry with the right person, to the right degree, at the right time, for the right purpose, and in the right way – that is not easy.*
>
> Aristotle (the Nicomacean Ethics)

So begins Daniel Goleman's book *Emotional Intelligence.*[1] The idea that emotional intelligence has a major role in determining your success in life has been around for thousands of years, but it is a relatively new concept for most Primary Care health professionals and it is a skill you will need to develop to thrive in the world of management. Traditional concepts of intelligence (IQ) concentrate on knowledge and cognitive skills; emotional intelligence (EQ) includes knowing what your feelings are and using them to make good decisions in life (See Box 12.1).

Self-awareness means recognising your feelings as they are happening. Your feelings are highly influenced by your personality and by your value system.

Box 12.1 The four areas of emotional intelligence.
- Self-awareness
- Self-management
- Social awareness
- Social skills

Consider the following situations:

> You are sitting in one of your first committee meetings of the Professional Executive Committee for your Primary Care Trust (PCT). The discussion has been going around in circles for the past five minutes; it is obvious to you what should be decided, why can't they decide?
>
> Another member of the committee is hogging the attention of the group, holding forth (with obviously limited expertise), and seemingly able to develop ideas 'on the hoof'. You feel you have the expertise to contribute but would like to have time to consider the implications. It seems so unfair . . .
>
> The nurse member of the committee makes disparaging remarks about lazy general practitioners shipping half of their workload onto nurses. She doesn't mean it as a personal remark, but you can't help feeling hurt by it . . .
>
> You joined the committee because you wanted to improve services to patients, yet this group seems more concerned with cutting costs . . .

You are aware of your emotions, feelings of irritation and frustration, perhaps of hurt, but where have they come from? The answer lies in the shape of your personality. We all have differently shaped personalities. There is not a right or wrong personality to have; differing personalities just work more or less effectively depending on the situation we find ourselves in.

Personality has been analysed in terms of four pairs of traits by the mother and daughter partnership of Kathryn Briggs and Isabel Myers,[2] dimensions that were originally described by Carl Jung.[3]

E or I	Extraversion or Introversion
S or N	Sensing or iNtuition
T or F	Thinking or Feeling
J or P	Judging or Perceiving

Box 12.2 (from co-contributor Julia Oxenbury) indicates typical behaviours exhibited by individuals of certain Myers–Briggs *preferences*.

Box 12.2 **Myers–Briggs personality preferences.**

Judgers	Perceivers
Make most decisions pretty easily	May have difficulty making decisions
Are serious and conventional	Are playful and unconventional
Pay attention to time and are prompt	Are less aware of time and run late
Prefer to finish projects	Prefer to start projects
Work first, play later	Play first work later
Want things decided	Want to keep their options open
See the need for most rules	Question the need for many rules
Like to make and stick with plans	Like to keep plans flexible
Find comfort in schedules	Want the freedom to be spontaneous
Seek closure	Go with the flow
Plan	Adapt as they go
Value neatness and tidiness	Are content with clutter

Extraverts	Introverts
Have high energy	Have quiet energy
Talk more than listen	Listen more than talk
Think out loud	Think quietly inside their head
Act then think	Think then act
Like to be around people	Feel comfortable being alone
Prefer a public role	Prefer to work behind the scenes
Can sometimes be easily distracted	Have good powers of concentration
Prefer to do lots of things at once	Prefer to focus on one thing at a time
Are outgoing and enthusiastic	Are self-contained and reserved
Enjoy groups	Enjoy 1:1

Sensors	Intuitors
Focus on facts and details	Focus on ideas and the big picture
Admire practical solutions	Admire creative ideas
Notice details and remember facts	Notice everything new or different
Are pragmatic - see what is	Are imaginative – see what could be
Live in the here-and-now	Think about future implications
Trust actual experience	Trust their gut instincts
Like to use established skills	Prefer to learn new skills
Like step-by-step instruction	Like to figure things out for themselves
Work at a steady pace	Work in bursts of energy
Prefer concrete information	Prefer abstract information

Thinkers	Feelers
Make decisions objectively	Decide based on their values and feelings
Appear cool and reserved	Appear warm and friendly
Are most convinced by rational arguments	Are most convinced by feelings
Are honest and direct	Are diplomatic and tactful
Value honesty and fairness	Value harmony and compassion
Take few things personally	Take many things personally
Tend to see flaws	Are quick to compliment others
Are motivated by achievement	Are motivated by appreciation
Are not put off by conflict	Avoid arguments and conflicts

The first example of interpersonal conflict described on page 144 is probably an example of the commonest form of interpersonal dispute or relationship difficulty. It occurs between individuals at either end of the Judging–Perceiving spectrum. *Judgers* tend to plan ahead and value structure and order. They are very goal orientated and would prefer to work first and play later; they like to complete projects and have things settled and decided. *Perceivers*, by contrast, seek openness and spontaneity, are flexible, and adapt as they go. They are much more easy going, like to start projects, but would prefer to play now and work will always be there for later! Conflicts arise when decisions have to be made. Judgers make decisions relatively more rapidly than do Perceivers and having made a decision they tend to move on. They see Perceivers as airy-fairy people unable to get things done. Perceivers, on the other hand, watch as Judgers rush headlong into things, making wrong decisions because they act too quickly and fail to consider all of the possibilities inherent in a situation.

In the second example, a conflict has arisen between the Extraversion–Introversion pair. This describes our attitude towards the world, what energises us. The *Extravert* (75% of the population) enjoys interactions and discussions with others in a group, as this helps them produce their best ideas. Extraverts tend to think out loud and can be annoyingly talkative. They change their behaviour according to the demands of this external world and so can comfortably fit in. *Introverts*, on the other hand, tend to behave in ways that have meaning for them; they enjoy thinking and reflecting, focusing inwards first before acting. Introverts need to understand a situation and what it means for them before they can make decisions about it and will often persist in following their own direction despite outside pressure.

The third pair in the type indicator is the Sensing–Intuition pair. This refers to how we prefer to take in information. *Sensors* (again 75% of the population) prefer facts and concrete information, they focus on the present, they are practical and realistic and value common sense. 'Why?' is the general mode of the *Intuitor*; they like to focus on the big picture, on what is possible. Intuitors value innovation and can be inspired and ground-breaking. As you can imagine, if you are in a strategy planning meeting and somebody is more interested in speculating on the meaning and relationship of ideas, it will be extremely annoying to the 'two feet firmly on the ground' Sensor.

Finally, we come to the Thinking–Feeling pair. This refers to how we evaluate information and make decisions. Consider the third example on page 144; the 'hurt' doctor, who has taken remarks personally. She is likely to be a *Feeler*, somebody who makes decisions based on values and these values act as a compass to determine the right course of action. She values harmony and relationships and is usually very tactful. The alternative is the *Thinker*, the person who decides on the basis of rational, logical analysis. Thinkers weigh up the evidence for a course of action, criticise the alternatives, and then make a decision logically, which can make them seem hard sometimes as opposed to the overemotional Feeler. I have deliberately chosen to label my Feeler as a woman; this is the only pair of traits that show a sex-related distribution – more women than men are feelers.

We have all developed a value system, however, and we use it to guide our actions. It is important to recognise your own values, because if you are forced to work in a system where they are compromised, you will feel stressed.

Try this at home

Keep a record of how you feel after interactions with different people (family, colleagues, friends, and patients) in different settings (at home, in the practice, at the PCT). You will probably find you have a set of scenarios similar to the ones described above. Reflect on these and try to analyse what it tells you about your personality traits.

Consider having your personality tested; the formal Myers–Briggs Test is probably the gold standard but may be too time-consuming and costly. An alternative could be the Keirsey temperament sorter.[4,5] Cross-reference your results with those of trusted colleagues and friends. Is this how they see you?

Self-esteem is the belief you have in yourself and your level of self-acceptance. It is a vital part of determining how you live your life and the depth of satisfaction you achieve from it. Self-esteem develops early in childhood and can be very difficult to change but not impossible and one needn't become trapped in a negative self-image; it is not a constant and ebbs and flows as you react to the environment and other people.

Consider the following two members of a Primary Care team who are faced with a major change in the way they work, perhaps the imposition of a new contract...

Person A
- Sees the changes proposed as a threat
- Feels tired at the thought of 'all that work'
- Doesn't believe they have the skills to be able to cope
- Feels other members of the team are and will be 'putting on them'
- Knows whatever they do won't be good enough for the others

Person B

- Sees the changes proposed as an opportunity
- Is enthused and energised by the thought of a new challenge
- Believes in their own ability to cope with the challenge and doesn't worry about the possibility of making a mistake
- Knows it will be a team effort with everybody contributing what they are able to
- Is happy to receive praise for good work done and positively feeds back to others
- Accepts negative criticisms and suggestions for change positively

There is obviously a huge difference in the self-esteem of our two team members and, consequently, there will be a huge difference in the way they are able to respond to the new challenges that face them.

Medical training for my generation (but hopefully less so now) was not conducive to a positive self-image. I can hardly remember any positive feedback; training seemed to be a process of ritual humiliation. But remember, it is possible to improve your self-esteem and the esteem of others close to you (but it takes some work).

You will now be in a position to recognise and respect your emotions. The next facet of emotional intelligence is realising that you don't have to respond to these feelings immediately; i.e. *self-management*. It is sometimes better to defer a judgement in an emotionally charged situation, to allow time for things to sort themselves out, so that eventually you will be able to express yourself in a way that reflects your own feelings whilst at the same time considering the feelings and emotions of others. Goleman cites the classic 'marshmallow' experiment conducted by Stamford psychologists in the 1960s with four-year-olds as illustrative of this point. The psychologists interviewed the children individually and offered them a choice; either they could have one marshmallow now or if they waited until the researcher had come back from running an errand they could have two. When the children were followed up 14 years later they found that this test was an amazing predictor as to how the children had done at school. The third that had been able to wait were more emotionally stable, better liked by their peers and their teachers, and still able to delay gratification in pursuit of their goals, which contributed powerfully to their intellectual potential.

Try this at home
Think back to when you were a child (or perhaps even now). What happened to your Easter eggs? What does it tell you about your self-regulation?

'Flow' is a term used for what we experience when performing at our peak, when we have a masterly control of what we're doing and are able to stretch beyond our former limits. What makes you 'flow'?

> *I was running a newly developed seminar on communication skills with medical students. I had carefully prepared the content; it was very interactive with lots of opportunity for positive feedback, so I was confident that it would be perceived as a good session. As the session progressed, things just seemed to be getting better and better; the group jelled, I was able to adapt the material I had produced to their particular needs, and the positive feedback meant that they all contributed more than they usually did. The session seemed to be over in a flash . . .*

What was happening here was that I was experiencing flow. My emotions were positive, energised and aligned to the task in hand. I had forgotten about everyday life and worries, I was completely concentrating on the work and my resulting performance was better than anything I had anticipated. Flow is a wonderfully rewarding, fulfilling feeling and it motivates you to 'want to do more'.

Experiencing flow will enable you to remain positive even in adversity, so you can take the initiative and seize opportunities as they present themselves.

Try this at home

To experience flow

- Choose a task you're extremely skilled at: it could be work-based, for example consulting with patients, or home-based – playing squash, playing the piano, painting a picture.
- Engage in it at a level that slightly taxes your ability.
- Intentionally focus sharp attention to the task in hand.
- Concentrate like mad . . .

Did it work?

Perhaps not completely this time, but if you persevere . . .

With regards to the remaining competencies of EQ, the contribution of social-awareness and 'social skills' is beyond the scope of this chapter, but knowing yourself better will, and this perhaps goes without saying, do wonders for your 'empathy'.

Try this at home

- Develop the habit of reflection (it's what the bath is for!). Identify what went well (particularly if you experience flow) and what qualities you used to make it happen. Conversely, identify situations that were difficult and use them to inform your development plan.
- Practice positive feedback. If you see something being done well, feed it back. Significant event audit offers a wonderful opportunity for the whole team to develop a 'no blame culture' and praise what was done well in addition to looking at systems to prevent the adverse event happening again.
- In negative feedback criticise the behaviour rather than the person. Describing somebody as rude or difficult is unhelpful. It is much better to say, 'When you said... it wasn't helpful, perhaps you could try wording it like this...'

Career orientation and development

You work best when you are engaged in something you care about that gives you pleasure. You need to choose work that nourishes you and gives you opportunities to grow and develop yourself and to flow.

As mentioned before, certain personalities find it easier to thrive in certain situations. Keirsey[5] divided personality types into four main groups that he called 'Temperaments' (see Box 12.3).

Box 12.3 **Keirsey's four temperaments.**
1. **Rationals** are motivated by the need for knowledge and competency, valuing the theoretical and powers of the mind
2. **Idealists** are motivated by a need to understand themselves and others, valuing authenticity and integrity
3. **Artisans** are motivated by a need for freedom and need to act, valuing living for the moment
4. **Guardians** are motivated by a need to be responsible in whatever social group they are in, valuing tradition

If your personality falls into the group he calls *Rationals*, then you would thrive in roles that have a strategic and planning function; working with the PCT on various committees would play to your strengths. Equally, your thinking skills would be invaluable in an academic department of Primary Care, participating in research.

Idealists can use their diplomacy to advantage when working with people.

Primary Care should seem like a very comfortable habitat for you, particularly in a teaching role. Alternatively, your personality is ideally suited to working as an appraiser or Continuing Professional Development tutor, encouraging others to develop professionally.

Artisans could find partnership in a practice very restrictive and they would be ideally suited to a portfolio career, particularly one in which their decision making skills would be fully utilised. Working as a Practice Nurse would not be playing to your strengths, but district nursing would be.

Finally, we come to the 'pillars of society'. *Guardians* would thrive as a senior partner or lead nurse. They tend towards pragmatism. A new contract would be manipulated to their own advantage, seen as an opportunity to increase their service provision to patients and to increase the practice income.

There are essentially two ways to determine your career development; either you can drift and let circumstances and opportunities determine your path or you can choose direction. Covey[6] believes that the first habit one has to acquire to become personally effective is to be proactive; i.e. to accept responsibility to make choices (see Box 12.4). This ability to make choices about the direction to take is essential for the development of positive self-esteem.

It is necessary, though, when choosing your career direction to be aware of where your priorities lie. For many mothers with young children the absolute priority is with the family and many women feel that running a family with a career is impossible. The secret here is to be flexible. Both the flexible career scheme and the GP Retainer scheme allow you to work with a limited commitment at times when you can organise childcare. Alternatively, think laterally: it may be impossible currently to consider working during the day, but how about working two evenings a week for one of the out-of-hours services when your partner can provide the child care? These organisations are increasingly looking for professionals to work from home providing a triage service.

I believe that General Practice in its current form is unsustainable; it feels like all demand and no reward. A good antidote to these feelings is to develop an

Box 12.4 **The seven habits of highly effective people (Stephen Covey).**
1. Be proactive
2. Begin with the end in mind (develop a vision)
3. Put first things first (prioritise)
4. Think win/win (in your interactions with others)
5. Seek first to understand then be understood
6. Synergise
7. Sharpen the saw (refresh yourself)

alternative interest. If you decide on a professional interest then use your appraisal to develop your ideas further. Appraisal (see Chapter 3) offers a wonderful opportunity to discuss your personal development with a trusted colleague. The appraiser has no personal 'axe to grind' (unlike a spouse or partner); they can help you develop a vision as to where you want to develop, which may contain both short- and long-term goals, and help you produce an achievable development plan. However, it is important to realise that life never proceeds along completely predictable pathways and your development plan is not 'set in stone'. If you want to develop a special interest in dermatology, for example, approach the PCT about opportunities for GPs or nurses with a special interest. Broadcast your talents; describe the improvement in service to patients that you will make; how could they resist you? Covey suggests that if two effective people work together they will synergise, i.e. the result is greater than the constituent parts, so find your allies who want to develop the service with you. If your plans don't fit in with those of either your practice or the PCT, don't despair; now is the time to think laterally and persevere (use your EQ). My GP colleague who was unable to develop her dermatology interest saw an advertisement for a clinical assistant in genitourinary medicine a few weeks later. She now has an absorbing alternative interest that contains an amazingly high proportion of dermatology.

Try this at home
Participate in appraisal

Work–life balance

Effectiveness requires a balance between the various roles in your life, your health, and your family. Can success in one aspect of your life make up for failure in another? One suspects not. It is very easy to take the relationships that matter most to us for granted. We kid ourselves that the wife and kids will understand when we come home grumpy from a demanding day at work responding to others' needs. They don't; they have needs too and look to you to help provide for them. Covey, again, introduces the idea of an emotional bank account. He uses it to describe the amount of trust and safeness in a relationship that is built up over time from small deposits of support and attention. Our most constant relationships need the most constant deposits and you need to be there to make them. To cope with the demands of our profession we need to be fit: physically, mentally, and spiritually. We need to find enjoyable ways to enable this to happen, preferably ways that enable us to experience flow.

Living fully who you are is connected to the art of medicine.[7]

References

1. Goleman D. *Emotional Intelligence*. London: Bloomsbury, 1996.
2. Myers IB, Myers PB. *Gifts Differing: understanding personality type*. Palo Alto, CA: Davies-Black, 1995.
3. Jung CG. *Psychological Types*. Princeton: Princeton University Press, 1971.
4. www.keirsey.com
5. Keirsey D. *Please Understand Me: temperament, character, intelligence*. Del Mar, CA: Prometheus Nemesis, 1998.
6. Covey SR. *The Seven Habits of Highly Effective People*. London: Simon and Schuster, 1989.
7. McMullen B. Emotional intelligence. *BMJ* 2003; **326(suppl)**: s19–20.

Chapter 13

Time Management

David Haslam

 KEY MESSAGES
- Prioritise
- Delegate
- Appreciate
- Switch off

Your time is precious. If you want to save yourself half an hour of valuable time straight away, this chapter can be summarised in the following words: prioritise, delegate, appreciate, and switch off.

'Time management' is one of those buzz phrases that has made its way into all of our lives over the last few years. For reasons that sometimes elude me, we are all much busier than we used to be, or at the very least we all feel that we are much busier, and efficient use of time has become more and more important. The phrase 'cash rich, time poor' has become a potent way of describing many professionals for whom time is the one thing that they really lack.

A quick search on the internet currently reveals a mere one million and fifty thousand websites devoted to this topic. To look at these for just one minute each would take a mere one hundred days of undisturbed time – with sleeping and eating not allowed. Amazon.com sells 2301 books on time management. There is clearly a real hunger for information and guidance, but as with all medical treatments, you know full well that if there was a guaranteed successful answer there would be one very famous book, and one very well-read website. The plethora of resources hints not that there are countless experts but that there are countless suggestions – which is not quite the same thing.

But I will endeavour to make this chapter worth your while. Life is much too short to waste your time reading articles that won't help, in the same way that it is much too short for bad wine or boring music. So, lesson one – if this doesn't seem to be helping, prioritise by moving on.

First, though, a simple exercise. Do you know – really know – why you get stressed? Most of us assume that it is the pressure of the job, the constant potentially life or death decisions, the paperwork, the state of the NHS. But can you be sure?

A simple way to find out is to complete a stress diary. Whilst this may sound like the very worst form of Californian psycho-babble, it is in fact an invaluable way of finding out where the real stresses in your life are coming from. The technique is simple.

Try this at home

For a period of 2–3 days, every hour, on the hour, record your stress level, and your happiness level on a scale of 0–10

The figures are relatively meaningless – don't agonise over them – just use your gut instinct. 0 could mean zero stress/total relaxed bliss, whilst 10 could be the worst stress you have ever felt.

Ignore the numbers, except when there is a change of 2 or more points from one hour to the next. When this happens, write down why – honestly, briefly, quickly.

I have used this simple exercise with many patients, but more importantly I have used it with many doctors. Almost without exception, the number one trigger of increasing stress and decreasing happiness turns out to be a time pressure. As an example, here is my own personal chart, taken from several years ago when I was feeling particularly stressed, and blaming the Conservative Government, my partners, NHS bureaucracy, and any other scapegoat that came to mind. So what did it reveal?

Time	Stress Score	Happiness Score	Reason for Change
8 a.m.	7	5	
9 a.m.	9	3	Taking kids to school. Nothing ready as ever
10 a.m.	6	5	Doing surgery
11 a.m.	5	5	
12 noon	6	7	Doing visits. Sunny day
1 p.m.	9	4	Late for lunch. Waiting for nurse – supposed to be doing joint home visit for leg ulcer

To my complete astonishment, it wasn't life and death decisions that made me stressed. It wasn't NHS reforms, or a paranoid feeling that I was seeing more visits than my partners. It was being late for my lunch, or the children being late for school. For some bizarre reason I had promised myself that I would stop for a brief lunch at home at 1 o'clock – to listen to the news whilst I had a sandwich. But this simple desire had actually become a problem rather than a benefit. Once spotted, it was easy to deal with, but I would never have predicted this if I hadn't done the exercise. Try it. You will be surprised, too.

Prioritise

You are never, ever going to get everything done. On the day that you die, there will almost certainly be letters left unwritten, books that you won't have read, and places that you won't have been. Accept it. You won't do everything, so make sure you do the things that you really need to do. This chapter focuses on time management as it applies to our lives in Primary Care. On the day you retire, there will still be outstanding papers in your in-tray. But the world will survive. The graveyards are full of indispensable people.

Patient care

In British General Practice we are generally superb at using time effectively and efficiently. Doctors in most other countries look at the number of patients that we see each day, and the length of time we have to offer each patient, with incredulity. Half-hour consultations are common elsewhere and unheard of in the UK. Part of the whole success of the NHS results from this astonishing time effectiveness, but trying to do too much too quickly is a recipe for stress and ineffectiveness, as well as speed and efficiency.

Caring for patients takes time and energy. The most routine of surgeries can reveal sudden, unexpected problems, which can completely throw your thought processes and disrupt your planning. Primary Care is an exceptionally difficult place to work – the potentially overwhelming nature of the different problems that face us can be astonishing. At the start of every day you can have no idea at all of what will have arisen by the end.

> At the end of a relatively routine consultation, a 55-year-old patient of mine who was on Tamoxifen for her breast cancer suddenly asked me if she could be considered for hormone therapy to induce her to become fertile again so that she could bear a surrogate child for her infertile diabetic daughter. She knew the therapy would cause her cancer to flare up and kill her, but, as she said, 'What better legacy could I leave than a child for my only daughter – the one thing that she truly craves.' And at the end of an apparently routine consultation she wanted my advice on the financial, practical, moral, legal, and ethical aspects of this idea.

I would be astonished if you have had an identical case to my middle-aged woman with breast cancer, but you too will have had problems that tested you to your limits, that you will never forget, and that were entirely unpredictable. Indeed, there are only a very few laws of General Practice, but the most infallible is:

The only entirely predictable thing about General Practice is that it is unpredictable.

So, accept the fact that on almost every single day of your professional life you will find that unpredictable things will happen. Sometimes they will be major – such as the patient who needs a mental health section in the middle of a busy surgery. Sometimes they will be much more minor, even trivial. But they will happen. In most surgeries there will be at least one patient who needs considerably longer than their allotted time. And if you know that something unpredictable is likely to affect your day, plan for it.

In my morning surgeries, I always have a 30-minute coffee break. This means, of course, that my morning surgery finishes 30 minutes later than it would otherwise have done, but the 30-minute gap allows for catching up when the unpredictable happens, as it inevitably will. If I'm called out to an urgent visit, if a consultant needs to speak to me on the phone, if a complex case needs dealing with at length there and then, this 30-minute buffer allows the day to continue without being totally disrupted. And on some astonishing days I even manage to get a cup of coffee.

It is also well worth remembering that not everything has to be done now. There are medical emergencies that need to be completely sorted on first presentation – crushing chest pain, suicidal middle-aged patients, and acute psychosis being but three – but many problems genuinely are too complex to deal with in a single consultation. Some physical problems need you to take time over considering the differential diagnoses and arranging investigations, and need review and re-examination. Accept this, explain to the patient that you are taking their case seriously and want to do the very best for them and the consultation will have a much better outcome than rushing to an outcome today. As in so much else, the way in which you explain this makes all the difference to the doctor–patient relationship. When faced with a hugely complex problem, particularly an emotional one, you may feel you need to see the patient again. A curt 'I'm too busy to deal with all this today' will create antibodies. A positive 'I'm really glad you've raised this with me today. It must be quite difficult to get that all off your chest. I want to give you the time this deserves' will create appreciation, and indeed recognition that you are really taking them seriously.

Without a doubt, for many long and complex emotional problems, telling the doctor can be quite exhausting for the patient. Indeed, much that you say and talk about in the rest of the consultation may well not be taken in. Fixing a follow-up a few days later can frequently make for a much more effective consultation, and effectiveness ultimately saves time.

Educational meetings

Whether you are attending meetings as a speaker or a delegate, you need to choose your topics carefully. Don't attend simply out of a sense of guilt or duty. Attend because it will be a sensible use of your time.

Some years ago, one particular educational meeting caused me to stop and think and examine my priorities. I had been asked to speak about stress in General Practice, one of my favoured topics, at Borchester Postgraduate Centre. I looked in my diary, saw with great relief that I was already busy that evening at Ambridge Young Practitioners Workshop, and so said – with a happy heart – that no, I couldn't manage the meeting.

I considered myself reasonable and sensible until I realised that if my diary had been empty that evening and I had been spending an evening at home with my wife, dog, and a glass of chilled Sauvignon Blanc, then I would have probably felt duty bound and obliged to say 'yes' to the request. A logical outside observer might deduce that this means that I would rather spend my time going to meetings than spending time with my wife, dog, and chilled white wine. This is, of course, nonsense.

I can be fairly certain that the same problem applies to you. An empty slot in your diary makes you feel under pressure to attend meetings. A filled slot makes you say 'no' with total relaxation. The answer: put time for relaxation in your diary. And give it priority. If someone asks you to be at a meeting at that time and you would be relaxing, you should only agree to go if you genuinely would value the meeting more than your sanity, your relaxation, and your life.

Journals

It has been calculated that the output of research in medical scientific journals is now so huge that if you are a truly conscientious reader, and every day read two papers in an attempt to keep up to date, at the end of 12 months you will be approximately 400 years behind schedule in your reading.

So reading everything is not possible. Many of us still pile up the journals and newspapers that arrive through our letterboxes in the corner, promising that we will read them when we have the time. And the pile gets larger and larger, nagging you all the while, until you eventually hire a skip, throw them away, and start again.

Be honest. Decide what you will read, and what you won't. Throw the rest away. Choose maybe one of the weekly papers (unless you enjoy reading them all), the *BMJ*, the *BJGP*, and any other – such as the *Practitioner* or *Update* that you feel is really useful – and then ditch the rest. If there is anything really important, you will hear it again elsewhere. The world will still keep turning if you don't allow the piles of unread paper to dominate your office. Take control.

When it comes to guidelines, be realistic. Taking on board everything that experts tell us that that we should be doing in General Practice is quite impossible. In an excellent paper as long ago as 1998, Arthur Hibble and his colleagues looked at all the guidelines that were facing GPs, and found 243 single-page and 195 two-page guidelines.[1] There were, however, 160 guidelines that were more than ten pages long, including 25 presented as booklets or large folders. About 60% of the guidelines had been produced locally, of which 50% had been produced by local trusts and 30% by GPs. In total they found 855 different guidelines, which resulted in an astonishing pile of paper 68 cm high and weighing 28 kg.

Don't let this accumulation of paper, books, journals, and guidelines threaten you, nag you, and demoralise you. It is NOT possible to read everything. Clear prioritisation is the solution.

Administration

If you enjoy the administrative side of practice, then please revel in your enjoyment. If you don't, then delegate (see below). Doctors and managers should be symbiotic. We should bring our clinical skills to our practices, and provide the clinical direction. Managers bring distinct and essential management skills. Doctors are too frequently obsessed with keeping their hand on the tiller of every single development. Unless you enjoy it, remember that it isn't what you were trained for. You don't have to do everything.

But whatever you choose to do in the administration of your practice, you will still be faced with paperwork. So here are a few basic suggestions for surviving the paperwork mountain:

- One-touch paper handling is essential. When a document arrives, whenever you can you need to read it, file it, or bin it. Now. Putting it on a 'to be read later' pile will simply create guilt and delay. Only do this if there really is no possible alternative.
- Don't waste your time even glancing at junk mail.
- Devise a simple practice system in which everyone knows where important incoming documents are kept. The ideal is perhaps scanning into a practice intranet, but a central filing system for hard copies can be equally effective. If every doctor keeps separate documents in his or her own room, the recipe will be chaos and hours spent searching.

Delegate

In the course of any given surgery in your practice, you will have seen large numbers of patients, needed to arrange investigations and referrals, required forms to be filled in, had phone calls to be made, patients to be contacted, results to be analysed, and who knows what other activities triggered by the unpredictable events described above.

You can't do it all. If you have just started a new practice and only have a very few patients, then doing everything might be an option, but for most of us it just is not possible. So don't try. Learn to delegate. Support your team. Advise, encourage, listen, share. Keeping your hands on everything is a mark of insecurity – trust your team, and let go.

Like all skills, delegation takes practice. At the beginning of your career, you may find it difficult to trust the person you delegate tasks to, largely because you don't quite trust yourself. But few things are more necessary to your survival as a GP than being able to share the load. And this may come as a shock, but the people you delegate to may actually do the job better than you would do it yourself.

Appreciate

And then, when you have mastered the art of letting go of tasks to your team members, make sure that you tell them when they do things well, and not just when things go wrong. This isn't just good person management, and simple humanity, it is highly time-efficient, too – a valued team will work together more than a criticised one. This might be a short paragraph, but it is core to everything else that you do. Because if your team doesn't feel valued, you won't feel able to delegate. And if you can't delegate, you won't be an effective GP.

Switch off

If you have done your best in your day's work, have delegated where you can, and have appreciated those who are working with you, then switch off. Stop. Parkinson's Law really does apply in General Practice even more than it does in all other aspects of life – work really does expand to fill the time available. You will often gain nothing from working for hour upon hour upon hour. You will become less effective, more exhausted, and will seriously risk burnout.

Burnout is the ultimate manifestation of stress, and is a term that originally came from rocket science – where a rocket has completely burnt out its fuel and is thus totally useless – but still appears to be moving forward and doing its job. This may sound familiar. Looking after yourself is essential, and that means stopping work and relaxing.

Finally, a few more simple time management tips.

- If you agree to do something – give a talk, write an article, contribute a chapter on time management – then it will take just as much work if your deadline is six months away as if the deadline is tomorrow. Don't let distance distort your planning. Even an elephant looks tiny in the distance.
- Talking of elephants – remember the old saying about eating an elephant sandwich. You don't try eating it all at once; you just take it a bite at a time. Complex tasks, including complex clinical problems, can be seen in just the same way.
- Remember that the perfect is the enemy of the good.
- Time creation is rarely possible but not impossible. When my children were young they slept dreadfully. Every morning I would get up with them at 5.30 in the morning to allow my wife to sleep on. To my surprise, I discovered that I didn't miss those morning hours in bed, and for several years, even after the children were morning sleepers, I got up early to write. With astonishment, I realised that one extra hour a day – in my case from 6 to 7 a.m. – equates to nearly two extra months of working time each year (based on a 40-hour working week). It was a quite extraordinary realisation, and using this time allowed me to write a weekly column in the GP press and a dozen or so books, without it impinging on my ordinary working day. But if you really do need your sleep, please don't try this method of time creation.
- Finally, remember that the old cliché 'If you want to get something done, ask a busy person' is true partly because some people do indeed use time better and more effectively, but largely because busy people often don't know how to say 'no'. So say 'no' more than you do now. It may come as a shock, but the world won't come to an end. Enjoy the time you save.

References
1. Hibble A, Kanka D, Pencheon D, Pooles F. Guidelines in general practice: the new Tower of Babel? *BMJ* 1998; **317**: 862–863.

Further reading
Amazon.com sells 2301 books on time management, or you could finish that novel . . .

Chapter 14

Problem Solving and Decision Making

Roger Neighbour

 KEY MESSAGES

- 'Thinking outside the box' is the key to effective problem solving.
- Decision making is problem solving in a 'big picture' context.
- To be effective, a model of the problem solving process should take account of human psychology, and suggest how the various stages are to be achieved.
- Strategies for solving clinical problems can be applied (with all their benefits and pitfalls) to other categories of problem.
- Creativity in problem solving can be stimulated by, for example, brainstorming, mind-mapping, or lateral thinking techniques.
- Recognising 'meta-dimensions' to problem solving and decision making will help to understand how problems arise and decisions are made.

If you are hoping, after reading this chapter, to know how to solve problems more effectively and to make better decisions, stop before the section called 'That's all very well, but . . .' By then you may feel sure that for every problem there is a simple solution, and that there is a straightforward process for arriving at it. To read further may discourage you; for the truth is, as Umberto Eco put it, that 'for every complex problem there is a simple solution, and it's wrong'. Most problems in our clinical and professional worlds are, like people, complicated and messy. Most decisions have to be made on the basis of incomplete or incompatible data, and rational thought plays a smaller part in the process than we might hope.

This chapter is an armchair gymnasium for the problem solving faculty. GPs are professional problem solvers and decision makers, used to dealing with complexity and uncertainty. The more ways you have of thinking about problems and decisions, the more likely you are to come up with the best one when it's needed. Flexibility – 'thinking outside the box' – is the key to effective problem solving. As someone said, 'If you always do what you've always done, you'll always get what you've always got.'

It is worth briefly considering the differences between problem solving and decision making. There is clearly an overlap, both being a search for the most advantageous option in uncertain or hazardous circumstances. Problem solving tends to be a focused, single-issue, short-term, and solitary activity; the parameters of a 'successful' solution are either specified in advance or will be clearly recognised once achieved – a diagnosis made, a danger averted, a target reached. Decision making is more often a shared process, touched with issues of responsibility and accountability, and worked out within a longer timescale. Whether or not the outcome of decision making – a choice made, a plan agreed, a programme drawn up – is successful may not be known until events have moved on and evidence has been accumulated. The skills required for problem solving tend to be cognitive and *intra*personal ones – shrewd analysis combined with creative imagination. Decision making, by contrast, emphasises strategic thinking, and *inter*personal skills – collaboration, the ability to work in groups and to take an overview, to see 'the big picture' as well as its component factors. Effective decision making requires the capacity to see how an array of contributory problems is hierarchically nested within an overarching goal. Decision making is problem solving within a context.

> **'If you always do what you've always done . . .'**
> 20-year-old Duane registered recently with the practice of Drs Firmhand, Softy, and Newbody. He consulted Dr Firmhand, telling him that he was dependent on DF118 (dihydrocodeine) and requested a regular prescription for this drug, without which he said he would be driven to obtain supplies on the black market. Dr Firmhand refused, saying that he never prescribed for addicts. The next day Duane consulted Dr Softy with the same request. Dr Softy agreed to prescribe 70 tablets a week, provided Duane attended the surgery regularly for support and monitoring. The following week, however, Dr Softy was on holiday, so Duane came to see Dr Newbody.
>
> Dr Newbody considered it wasn't her place, as junior partner, to question Dr Softy's policy. Moreover, when Duane told her that he needed extra tablets to prevent withdrawal symptoms, she felt sufficiently intimidated by him to agree to double his supply of medication. When Dr Softy returned from holiday, Dr Newbody mentioned the increase to him. Dr Softy felt remorseful to have so badly underestimated Duane's needs. Dr Firmhand, overhearing their discussion, said this merely confirmed his view that there was no point trying to help drug addicts. Dr Newbody hoped Duane would not consult her again but suspected he probably would.
>
> Neither Dr Firmhand (who saw his rigidity as 'taking a principled

stand'), nor Dr Softy (who could sometimes be patient-centred to a fault),
nor Dr Newbody (who thought her role in the practice was to be
deferential to her seniors) recognised how attitudes that to them seemed
right were nonetheless perpetuating the problem.

Models of problem solving and decision making

Books on problem solving and decision making abound in airport bookstalls, and most include a flow chart 'how to do it' model. Model making – the simplification of complex processes to their symbolic essentials – is an established part of the medical toolkit, and is not to be decried. Models, like teddy bears, are toys to be played around with until the confidence to deal with real life is gained.

A basic model

Every doctor is familiar with the traditional 'medical model' for solving clinical problems:

- Take a systematic **history**
- Conduct a systematic **examination**
- Arrange **special tests**
- Arrive at the **diagnosis**
- Undertake appropriate **treatment**
- Arrange **follow-up**

The medical model is a special case of a widely taught problem solving paradigm:[1]

- Problem **presented**
- Problem **examined**
- Problem **defined**
- Solution **proposed**
- Solution **examined**
- Solution **implemented**

In other words:

When you encounter a problem . . .
mull it over until . . .
you're clear what the real problem is.
Then think what could be done about it . . .
decide what would be best, then . . .
do it!

Shorn of jargon and specialist context, a problem solving model like this does not at first sight seem much of an improvement on common sense. Certainly, it reminds us that being methodical is better than trial and error, and that thought should precede action. But in Primary Care the problems that tax us most are those that don't fit neatly into a linear analytic process. Our problems tend to be multi-stranded and to lie simultaneously within more than one domain. For example, trying to solve the problem, 'How will the practice gear up to meet national targets for diabetic care?' might, besides purely clinical considerations, involve: changing patterns of staffing levels; further education for nurses; the financial implications of extra staff and workload; interpersonal issues such as rivalries between colleagues; upgrading IT and administrative systems; and the ethical implications of emphasising the care of one group of patients to the possible detriment of others. A problem solving model, then, can be very useful in illuminating these issues.

To stand any chance of being realistic and useful, models of problem solving and decision making need two attributes. The first is that they should include some modelling of the human beings who are themselves both part of the problem and of the solution. Looking at the simple model described already, one would imagine that the people implementing it are logical, predictable, consistent, and transparent – in fact, computers. Problem solving would be much simpler if we were; machines (as Andy Warhol observed) have less problems. In reality, of course, as General Practice constantly reminds us, human beings are inconsistent and often illogical. They are opinionated, emotional, alternately noble and cantankerous, capable of rigidity and creativity in equal jaw-dropping measure. Advice to such fickle creatures on how to solve their difficulties will fail if it ignores their psychology.

The second crucial requirement of a useful model is that it should not only set out the stages of problem solving in sequence; it must suggest how each sequential stage is to be achieved. A good model addresses process as well as task.

The following are models that have tried to incorporate elements of 'the who and the how'.

Some refinements

Options, Implications, Choice. Effective patient-centred consulting includes a phase where doctor and patient jointly consider how the presenting problem is to be managed. The trilogy of options, implications, and choice (OIC) forms a convenient mnemonic. The OIC framework prompts discussion along the lines of, 'We could do A, B, or C. If A, this might happen; if B, that; if C, the other. Which seems to be the best?' It serves as an antidote to the easy escape offered by 'Doctor knows best', and reminds both parties to consider all options and think them through before settling on a course of action. The very vagueness of OIC is its strength, allowing it to be applied more generally beyond the consulting room. It places responsibility for the outcome firmly upon the problem solvers. Creativity and experience are needed to generate options; imagination to anticipate their consequences; and co-operation and commitment to implement the agreed plan.

SWOT. SWOT – Strengths, Weaknesses, Opportunities, Threats – is another problem solving framework that originated within the business management world. An organisation (or indeed an individual) confronting a problem might undertake a SWOT analysis, brainstorming internal resources under the Strengths and Weaknesses headings, and external circumstances under Opportunities and Threats. The suspension of criticism necessary for brainstorming encourages creativity, which subsequent discussion can, if skilfully conducted, channel into decisions and action plans.

Risk–benefit analysis. A SWOT analysis may suggest fresh options as possible solutions to a problem, but (as the OIC model reminds us) the implications of each must be evaluated. One way of doing this is to weigh the benefits of an option against its risks. Often this is done subliminally, almost intuitively. With complex or high-stakes problems, however, possible courses of action may be systematically rated along the two dimensions of foreseeable risk and expected benefit.

- Low-risk, low-benefit options can probably be discarded, or at least settled for only as a last resort.
- High-risk, low-benefit options are clearly best avoided, or a defence against them put in place.
- A low-risk, high-benefit option, if one exists, seems attractive. Remember, though, that if a thing looks too good to be true, it probably is.
- The high-risk, high-benefit option is the most challenging and therefore (possibly) the most attractive. At the very least, this is the one to research most thoroughly.

How a person or an organisation weights risk against benefit is a reflection of many factors, most of them psychological, and in particular of the prevailing value system. As Robert McKee, a noted Hollywood screenwriter, is fond of observing, 'Values are revealed by the choices we make under pressure.'

Importance vs. urgency. Good strategic decision makers can differentiate between *important* problems and *urgent* ones, and in so doing establish priorities (see Table 14.1). Lancing the carbuncle on the neck may be urgent, but controlling the patient's blood glucose is ultimately more important. Although it

Table 14.1 **Priority setting by importance and urgency.**

	Important	Not important
Urgent	*Do this first!*	
Not urgent		

sounds obvious, many problems are more difficult than they need be because the wrong problem is being tackled.

- Unimportant low-urgency matters can (to use a medical metaphor) take their place on the routine waiting list.
- Important low-urgency problems will always take priority over them in the admissions office.
- An urgent problem, even of low importance, requires same day attention.
- A problem that is both urgent and important is a crisis; an ambulance needs to be called.

Readers who have worked in A&E departments will have seen what happens when an 'important' case ties up resources needed by an 'urgent' one. One of the ironies of the NHS is that readers with management responsibilities will equally appreciate what happens when 'urgent' cases block facilities needed by 'important' ones!

Other types of problem solving in Primary Care

The medical model, for all that it is comprehensive and ultimately reliable, starts from an assumption that every known pathology could be the cause of the presenting problem, and systematically weeds out all except one of them. It takes little account of the doctor's experience, and makes inefficient use of time and resources. Other methods of clinical problem solving have been developed, and will translate readily enough to non-clinical settings. Roughly in order of increasing reliability, they include:

Habit

Some problems recur regularly and a solution that has always worked will probably continue to do so. The danger of relying on habit as a problem solving technique is that of 'If you always do what you've always done, you'll always get what you've always got'. If a practice always responds to a shortage of appointments by engaging a locum, it may never address more fundamental questions of workload.

Trial and error

Sloppy thinking of the 'If it's a rash, try a steroid cream' kind can be dangerous. The problem may deteriorate while ineffective solutions are tried that may in addition make things worse.

Probability

'Common things are common; the bird sitting on the fence is more likely to be a sparrow than a canary' can be a useful rule of thumb, but sometimes important outcomes depend on knowing a canary when you see one. Over-reliance on probability is (probably) the main reason serious conditions such as meningitis may be missed in General Practice. If relying on the balance of probabilities to solve a problem, make sure you have a 'safety net' in place. Ask yourself, 'How would I know if the solution wasn't working?'

Algorithms

Decision trees, in which a decision path through a complex issue is traced via a sequence of questions each with a 'yes or no' answer, have become popular in recent years. Clinical algorithms and protocols have proliferated, encouraged by the wish to achieve consistency of standards, to avoid dangerous errors, and to be able to delegate safely to less experienced colleagues. Sceptics (myself included) believe, however, that real people don't think in algorithms, which have no place for shortcuts based on experience or hunch, or for incorporating imprecise concepts such as 'maybe', 'sometimes', 'slightly', or 'it all depends'.

Pattern recognition

The Gestalt school of psychology is founded on the notion that we tend to perceive objects and situations 'all at once and all of a piece', recognising the sum of the parts before the individual parts themselves. This process is at work when we spot a patient's Parkinsonism as he walks through the door, or detect the depression underlying a request for some more headache pills. For problem solving by pattern recognition to be reliable, a sufficient repertoire of templates has to be acquired by experience. As someone said, 'To a man with a hammer, an awful lot of things look like nails.'

Hypothesis testing

GPs are no longer ashamed to admit that, in real life, we frequently abandon the formal medical model in favour of a cyclical method of decision making, where-by we make tentative assessments on the basis of incomplete data and act on them, but with the proviso that the original hypothesis will be modified in the light of subsequent developments or additional information. The teenager's sore throat is probably tonsillitis, so we prescribe penicillin. But it persists, and the axillary glands are tender, so we revise the provisional diagnosis to glandular fever. We're not surprised when she gets a rash – but it's urticarial, so more likely to be a penicillin allergy. Problem solving by hypothesis testing represents a practical compromise between formal logic, experience, algorithmic thinking, the efficient use of time, and working with incomplete data.

Decision making

Remember that decision making is just a special case of problem solving – problem solving within a particular context (such as a practice) and as part of a particular 'big picture' (such as improving patient care). However, when an impending decision could impact upon some vital aspect of an organisation's effectiveness or viability, it is all the more important to invoke a systematic decision-making process such as the following:

Identify issue(s) to be decided
- Prioritise
- Think strategically
- Involve other people if appropriate

Undertake analysis of relevant factors
- Use SWOT, etc
- Undertake research
- Generate new ideas
- Reassess previous decisions
- Challenge assumptions

Evaluate options
- Pros and cons
- Risk–benefit analysis
- Predict outcomes
- Resource implications
- Safety-netting against possible problems

Make decision
- Ensure process has been sound
- Check support and dissent
- Secure commitment of others involved

Implement decision
- Draw up action plan, including timeframe
- Communicate to relevant parties
- Delegate
- Monitor and review

That's all very well, but . . .

If you wish to gain knowledge of a problem, begin with learning to see it in many different ways.

Leonardo da Vinci (1452–1519)

Problems worthy of attack
Prove their worth by biting back.

Piet Hein (b. 1905)

Models and prompts such as those discussed earlier can provide a sense of focus and direction for our attempts at problem solving. However, even the most comprehensive model is at best a recipe; it is neither the ingredients nor the finished dish. People think analogically, not digitally. They have private thoughts as well as public, hidden agendas and hidden talents as well as acknowledged ones. They get mental blocks, and sometimes can't see the wood for the trees. They can be co-operative and creative but not always on demand. Formal schemes of decision making risk overlooking human idiosyncrasies while at the same time inhibiting creative thinking that goes 'outside the box'. The philosopher Bertrand Russell put his finger on it:

Everything is vague to a degree you do not realise till you have tried to make it precise.

Solving the wrong problem

Dr Softy and Dr Newbody agreed that their main problem dealing with Duane was a clinical one; although they were willing to help him, they felt they did not know enough about the most appropriate therapeutic and management strategies. So they arranged a meeting with a Community Psychiatric Nurse (CPN) with experience in addiction problems. The CPN advised them about dosage regimes and the importance of making a contract and setting boundaries with Duane, and offered ongoing support.

However, Dr Firmhand refused to have any further contact with Duane, and was annoyed when a receptionist inadvertently booked Duane in to see him. The receptionist burst into tears, explaining afterwards that a nephew of hers also had drug problems, and she therefore had a soft spot for people like Duane, who, she said, were often badly treated by doctors. Duane, who was still in the waiting room, heard these exchanges and smiled to himself.

Following this incident, Dr Firmhand drew up revised guidelines for the booking of emergency appointments, and asked Drs Softy and

> *Newbody in future to make sure that one of them was always available to see Duane. They said they could not give this guarantee, and criticised Dr Firmhand for what they considered his high-handed behaviour.*

Look back at the general problem solving paradigm at the beginning of this chapter. Between steps 3 and 4 ('problem defined' and 'solution proposed') is a small but crucial conceptual gap. Where do ideas come from? How do we get from understanding the problem to generating possible solutions?

Is it not the case that the solution to a problem can 'just spring to mind', that we sometimes 'just come up with' a good idea, and that decisions often 'make themselves'? Clearly, unconscious or preconscious processes are at work alongside the rational intellect. Intuition cannot be rushed; if the roast potatoes aren't done, you can turn the oven up – but not with meringues. Yet flashes of insight are not simply a question of luck. There are ways to make them happen more predictably. As one professional golfer remarked, 'It's odd; the more I practise, the luckier I get.'

You will be familiar with *brainstorming* – allowing the free flow of ideas, whilst agreeing not to criticise or evaluate. *Mind-mapping*[2] takes the process several stages further, charting clusters of linked ideas that radiate out from a central prompt. In the resulting access of creative energy, unexpected and surprising new possibilities often emerge.

Edward de Bono, who introduced the phrase *lateral thinking* to the language,[3] coined the new word 'Po' as a thinking tool to break the confines of rigid or habitual thought patterns.[4] Po means neither yes nor no, or both yes and no, as in 'Is general practice a good thing? Po.' It can also be used as a stimulus to think laterally, as in 'Does a clock have two hands? Po, it can have three, or six, or none; or feet, or a voice.' Such apparently facetious or counterintuitive responses can serve as half-way stages to developing alternative designs of timepiece.

The 'meta-' dimension

'meta-' denoting something of a higher or second-order kind

New Oxford Dictionary of English

Speed is the rate of change of position; acceleration is the rate of change of the rate of change of position; i.e. 'meta-change'. We use language to talk about most things, but need 'meta-language' to talk about language itself. There is an important 'meta-dimension' to the issues we are currently considering. There are 'meta-problems' about problems, such as 'How do problems arise in the first place?', and 'meta-decisions' to be made about how we make decisions.

Meta-problems

How do problems arise? Many problems, of course, come about because circumstances over which we have no control have changed. But sometimes a problem is really just a difficulty that has been mishandled. Perhaps action was needed but not taken; e.g. reduced staff availability during holiday periods was not planned for. Or action was taken where none was needed; e.g. prescribing habit-forming benzodiazepines after a lovers tiff. Or action was taken at the wrong level; e.g. trying to solve alcoholism by prohibition.

A common but potentially disastrous pattern, when a solution we are convinced is right has been tried but has failed, is to persist with it even more determinedly. Bleeding – 'letting out the bad blood' – was once considered so obvious a remedy that some patients, repeatedly bled, died of exsanguination. Insomnia sufferers are often but mistakenly advised to stay up late 'to get properly tired'. The solution compounds the problem.

Some people are compulsive problem manufacturers. Some hidden agenda may cause them to undermine or sabotage something that is working perfectly well. Or a 'need to be needed' may drive them to create problems that they alone can solve. Or fear that their own inadequacy might be rumbled may lead to a flurry of displacement activity that they hope might pass for action. Remember the saying, 'If it ain't broke, don't fix it.'

Reframing. 'When is a problem not a problem? When it's an opportunity.' Behind this cliché is the sound idea that a problem, like a symptom, is a system's way of indicating the need for change. Achieving this shift in perception is as key a skill in management as it is in therapy, and is called 'reframing'. Reframing involves fundamentally altering the meaning attributed to a situation through changing the conceptual and/or emotional context (the 'frame') within which it is interpreted. The adrenalin rush of stage fright may seem to be 'an anxiety problem', to be treated with propranolol, but it can be reframed as a welcome sign that the body is gearing up for optimum performance. As with a symptom of psychosomatic illness, the key to reframing a problem is to ask, 'What is this so-called problem trying to tell us about the way we currently do things?'

'Attitudes about attitudes'

Disagreements over Duane's case brought to a head some underlying tensions between the three partners. Sensing a potentially serious rift, they agreed to meet one evening to try to decide a policy they could all be happy with.

They met at Dr Firmhand's house over a takeaway curry. The more relaxed atmosphere away from the surgery enabled them to speak more

> openly to each other about their different attitudes to difficult patients,
> and the various experiences that had shaped them. They were able to
> reframe their conflict over Duane as arising from poor communication
> with each other, and from not having enough respect for each other's value
> systems. Although they continued to have differing views about drug
> addicts, they found they were better able to tolerate these discrepancies,
> and could agree on arrangements whereby Duane's care, and the smooth
> running of the appointments system, would not be compromised.
>
> The meeting (as Dr Softy later put it) 'changed our attitudes about our
> attitudes'. Finding he could no longer play one doctor off against another,
> Duane settled into a regime of dose stabilisation and reduction.

Meta-decisions

How is it decided what needs to be decided? Who makes decisions about the decision-making process? How do those in authority derive their authority? Whose version of the 'big picture' is the one that prevails? How far is it acceptable to question the status quo?

Sooner or later, 'meta-questions' like these have to be addressed within any organisation. Sometimes, of course, the answers are laid down by contract or statute. But ultimately it is through 'meta-process' – the assumptions and

---

Try this at home

Think of a reasonably significant dilemma or decision currently facing you in your own personal or professional life; e.g. whether to take out a bank loan, or how to redistribute responsibilities in the light of a revised GP contract.

As a 'thought experiment', and using pencil and paper, systematically work through (in your imagination) the detailed decision-making model set out in this chapter.

After doing this, reflect on (i) what aspects of, or factors in, the problem have been highlighted by the exercise, and (ii) the extent to which it helps to have a formalised framework for addressing it.

Then try the following supplementary exercise, based on one of Edward de Bono's techniques for stimulating creativity. Think of all the ways in which the problem or its apparent solution resemble three random inanimate objects. For example, a wheel (aids movement, best if frictionless, needs a centre of rotation, etc); a ladder (requires a firm base, brings high objects within reach, climbing may induce vertigo); or a painting (beauty is in the eye of the beholder, may look better in a frame, could be an investment). See whether making these apparently irrational connections suggests any possibilities you had not previously considered.

ground rules about process that are usually taken for granted – that an organisation expresses its core beliefs and values. Decision makers can acquire their authority in various ways: by election, seniority, delegation, aptitude, force of personality, corruption, tradition. Authority, too, can be exercised in a variety of styles: by diktat or consensus, top–down or bottom–up, by issuing orders, or by explanation and persuasion. There are seldom clear-cut right or wrong meta-decisions; what is important is that meta-process can be identified, discussed, and, if necessary, challenged.

References

1. Royal College of General Practitioners. *The Future General Practitioner: learning and teaching.* London: British Medical Journal, 1972.
2. Buzan T. *The Mind Map Book.* London: BBC Books, 1993.
3. de Bono E. *Lateral Thinking: a textbook of creativity.* Harmondsworth: Penguin Books, 1977.
4. de Bono E. *Po: beyond yes and no.* London: Penguin Books, 1973.

Further reading

Ceserani J. *The Problem-solving Pocketbook.* Alresford: Management Pocketbooks, 2003.
Heller R. *Making Decisions.* London: Dorling Kindersley, 1998.
> *Convenient résumés of the received wisdom about problem solving and decision making.*

Kosko B. *Fuzzy Thinking: the new science of fuzzy logic.* London: Harper Collins, 1994.
> *Sadly, I have yet to see 'fuzzy logic' successfully incorporated into clinical algorithms (though we do it by instinct in everyday life). There is a research opportunity here.*

Watzlawick P, Weakland J, Fisch R. *Change: principles of problem formation and problem resolution.* New York: WW Norton and Company, 1974.
Watzlawick P. *The Language of Change: elements of therapeutic communication.* New York: Basic Books, 1978.
> *Two fascinating books from the Brief Therapy Center of the Mental Research Institute in Palo Alto providing insightful analyses of how people get themselves into trouble (and can get themselves out of it).*

Chapter 15

Project Management

Helen Alpin

 KEY MESSAGES

- Project management provides a framework to help you deliver your project successfully.
- Health care professionals can be successful project managers.
- Project management works on a cycle; you need to know where you are going, plan how you are going to get there, and then go, being prepared to modify and adapt as necessary.
- Projects often fail because of lack of commitment especially of resources; be realistic in what will be needed to succeed.
- Avoid project creep, be clear about what your project will and will not cover.
- At the end learn from the experience so that next time you can do it better.

This chapter will attempt to lead you through project management, giving you an understanding of what project management is, the skills that it requires, and the tools that it utilises. It will take you through the stages of projects using examples of common projects that may take place in Primary Care.

What is project management?

A project is a defined piece of work that leads to the outcome of something new being created within a timescale. Projects can range in size from small to large, can be simple or complex, and timescales will vary accordingly.

Project management is a method that utilises recognised tools to identify what resources (e.g. time, people, money) will be needed to achieve specified objectives in a controlled and structured manner within a given timeframe.

Skills for project management

Many health care professionals, including doctors, have never had any training in project management. For success, a project requires a manager responsible for delivery and leadership, and the lack of dedicated expertise is a common feature in projects that fail. Many people managing projects in Primary Care will still have their 'day job' to do, which makes the need for the knowledge and use of effective project management tools and techniques even more important.

Project management involves:

- planning and definition
- implementation and control.

Planning is aided by tools, charts, and management skills, but the ability to take action requires a leader.

A project manager must have leadership skills and the ability to plan, gain consensus, and communicate effectively. They must be able to guide, facilitate, negotiate, and co-ordinate with energy and enthusiasm, making the right decisions at critical stages. In some situations in Primary Care because of the time constraints of clinical staff, it may be appropriate to share the role of project manager between the practice manager or another member of the administrative team and a clinician, optimising skills, knowledge, and experience, and also making sure that key stakeholders are committed to the project.

The lifecycle of projects

It is helpful to think that a project has a lifecycle. There are many different examples of such lifecycles in different industries, what we need is one that works in health care, in primary health care. The simplest is a three-stage cycle: *planning, implementing* and *closing* (see Figure 15.1). A more complex cycle may have five or six stages: *conception, definition, planning, launch and execution, controlling,* and *closure*. It is important to think cyclically as, during a project, when things change, you may have to go back to the previous stage to adapt or amend things.

Getting an idea off the ground

Lots of good ideas remain just that. There are many things within Primary Care that we must do, some we should do, and some we would like to do. In fact, there is so much to do that unless we are efficient with our limited resources, we will never get beyond the 'must do's', which we often resent because of their imposition and the fact that frequently they are not our personal or organisational priorities.

So if you have a good idea, share it and canvass feedback. It is never too early to get people on board and this will also give you a chance to see if your idea is really something to go for, worth devoting time and energy to achieve. For example, your practice might need to develop or completely rebuild its premises

Figure 15.1 **Project management cycle**

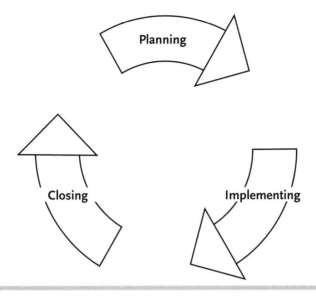

or need to recruit a new member of staff. The Primary Care Trust might require you to lead on the development of a new service, or on the implementation of an aspect of clinical governance. In a Department of Postgraduate General Practice you might be developing the Flexible Career Schemes, recruiting GP Tutors, supporting GP appraisal, or setting up a support structure for poorly performing professionals. Project management can help you achieve these objectives by utilising tools to identify what resources will be needed to succeed in a controlled and structured manner in a given timescale.

   Choosing the right idea to run with cannot be underestimated. Having made that decision you now need to think it through in a little more detail. You need to gain a better understanding of the overall objective, the specific goals that will be achieved, and the scope of the project before you move on to the planning stage. At this stage you also need to identify who the key players are, who is supporting this project, and where the funds are coming from. Once you know what you want to do, go and talk to people, explain what you are planning, engage them,

Try this at home
Identify the criteria for success
Before you start on your next project, just think of changes that have been successfully implemented in your organisation and conversely ones that haven't. Try and identify what factors are important to ensure a successful outcome and pitfalls to avoid.

and if you think that you will need them for part of your task, enlist their help. Start to identify who you need on your core project implementation team; for a small project it may just be you or one other key person. Listen and learn from others who may have done similar projects. Sources such as the Modernisation Agency website (www.modernnhs.nhs.uk) have a multitude of network contacts that may be able to help. Don't try and reinvent the wheel, save your resources for things that haven't already been conceived.

Box 15.1 **Key factors for success.**
- Choosing the right project
- Getting people on board
- Building a strong team
- Adequate resources, time, people, and money
- Commitment
- Leadership
- A vision of what will be achieved at the end of the project

---

As well as the overall aim for your project you will also have specific objectives. For instance, the overall aim for a project may be to rebuild the practice premises, but there will be a need to consider other specific issues such as by when, suitable for what, and within what specified budget. The objectives of your project should be *SMART*, that is Specific, Measurable, Achievable, Realistic, and Time-bound.

Box 15.2 **Define project goals.**
- To create something (e.g. a product, procedure, organisation, building)
- To be completed within a given budget
- To be completed within an agreed timeframe

The scope of your project needs to be defined; the scope is the size of the project, giving it boundaries, making it clear what it is going to deliver and what it will not cover. Beware of scope 'creep', that is the project becoming too broad and complex; it is often better to note additional sub-projects that may be needed to achieve related objectives rather than add them on so that the original project gets lost in the complexity.

Finally, at this stage you need to think about the constraints and risks of your project. The biggest constraint is likely to be your resources, especially money. The risks will vary in size and importance. However it is important even for a small project to think about the things that could derail your project and how you can either minimise these risks or deal with them if they arise.

Parkside Surgery is a five-partner practice in a suburban setting. Due to new housing in the area, the practice list has expanded recently and they now have around 8500 patients. The current surgery premises comprise a small three-bedroomed detached house, which has been adapted over the years. The reception area is too small and the treatment room and two consultation rooms are upstairs. The ground floor has been extended, but access remains poor and the practice is short of consultation rooms to house their expanding team. The partners have decided that they need new premises.

Let's look at this example, a common situation for many practices. From the outline given, the decision that new premises are needed seems to have been arrived at. The practice has tried to make do and mend, but it now has reached the stage where they need a new building. Here is a project and a chance to utilise project management skills and tools. The partners have an overall aim, which is to build new practice premises, but the scope of the project now needs to be defined. Are they going to include any new services? Will the practice team be reorganised as a result? Will they become a new training practice now that they have room? The list of possibilities is endless and the practice would be advised to confine themselves to building new premises, a project that will prove complex enough!

Thinking about the factors that will lead to success is helpful at this stage and a good way of engaging the practice team. Setting up a meeting to introduce the idea to practice staff, bringing together the core project team, and identifying the person who is going to lead on this project are all very important at this stage. Beware of dreaming; it is useful to share the constraint of the project before everyone gets carried away with ideas of helipads and roof gardens. Defining specific project goals is also important before moving on. For this particular project these may include: a target date for completion, that it will be completed within the specified budget, and that it should be fit for purpose; e.g. conforming to all current and anticipated legislation on accessibility and safety. Making a list of stakeholders and starting to engage them is also essential at this stage.

Planning

There are three components involved in the planning phase; the *task list*, the *schedule*, and the *budget*.

No matter how big or small the project (but more so if the project is large and/or complex), it is important to break the job down into tasks. Tasks are bite-sized chunks, cohesive pieces of work that split the project into manageable units. A task list will help determine the schedule for the project – e.g. identify in what order the work for the project should be carried out – and also helps in tracking, as it is easy to see when a specific task has been completed. Tasks can be carried out concurrently (i.e. at the same time) or they can run serially (i.e. one after another dependent on the completion of the previous task).

Once you have a list of necessary tasks and some breakdown, but not necessarily complete at this stage, of what each task involves, you need to be writing a bid in order to secure resources and support. For some projects part of your bid may be the business case behind your project. For other projects you may not need to write a bid but a project plan. The outline below should be helpful in constructing whatever document commits your plan to paper.

Writing a bid

After having the idea, agreeing that it is worth proceeding with, defining what the project is, and what it will achieve, the next questions are 'how' and 'with what' or 'who'. Sometimes a project will emerge out of the implementation of a resourced initiative so that funding may already be available, but often, for more original or creative ideas, resources will have to be found. Writing a bid is about selling your project and convincing others that it is worth investing in.

Like many documents, your bid will probably not be examined in great detail. So the document's appearance, the ease of access of information, and that it contains the information that potential sponsors will require are key issues. It is better to keep this type of document short, with supporting detail in appendices.

A bid should contain information under the headings in Box 15.3.

Evaluation should always be included in your bid. It is an important part of the process and is often forgotten if not planned for explicitly at the outset.

> Abbey Road Practice has just taken on a new partner who is very keen that the practice should become a training practice. The practice needs a significant amount of development before it will be acceptable as a training practice. The new partner has agreement from the other partners that they are keen for the practice to pursue this objective and she has the go-ahead to do whatever is necessary.

So, the new partner has a project. Here, the obvious leader is the partner herself and the core project team is probably just her and the practice manager. She has done the work of defining the project and has now reached the planning stage. She now needs to draw up the list of tasks that will need to be accomplished in order to gain training status. A series of tasks can be grouped together to form stages or steps in a project; for example, there will be a number of necessary

Box 15.3 **The information required in a project bid.**

Purpose of project
- *What is the general purpose of the project?*

Why should the project be done now?
- *Why is it opportune to do this project now?*
- *Putting the project in context; where does it fit in with other projects and objectives of the organisation?*

What benefits the project will bring
Plans of how it will be done
Resources that will be needed
- *Time, people, money, equipment, facilities, materials, information, and technology*

Budget
- *A breakdown of costs*

Risks
- *Assumptions and constraints*

Outcomes of the project
- *How will we know if we have been successful?*

Evaluation
Timescales

tasks to get all the records up to the required standard. Once these have been achieved a significant step in the project will have been achieved. At this stage she also needs to have written the project plan.

For simpler or smaller projects once you have a list of tasks you can move onto scheduling. Accurate, realistic, and workable scheduling is what makes a project tick. A schedule shows who is doing what, when they are supposed to be doing it, and how it all fits together in the bigger picture.

Gantt charts (see Figure 15.2) are a tool for showing a visual overview of project timelines. Usually, they have a list of dates at the top and a list of tasks down the left hand side. A bar on the Gantt chart shows the date each task begins and ends. Gantt charts can also show milestones, project meetings, and project reviews (e.g. financial, progress). Project management software can be helpful in producing a Gantt chart, as it allows easy modification and alteration.

The complexity and amount of information shown on Gantt charts is infinitely variable. What you need is a chart of your project's activities that helps you keep track of what is happening when, making it only as complicated as it needs to be. The amount of detail will be partially determined by the timescale that you choose, which depends on the duration of your project; for a project lasting a month you will need a daily chart, for a project lasting six months, a weekly chart. Some activities are dependent on each other; these interdependencies can be shown by additional lines, as shown in the diagram.

Figure 15.2 **A Gantt chart schedule**

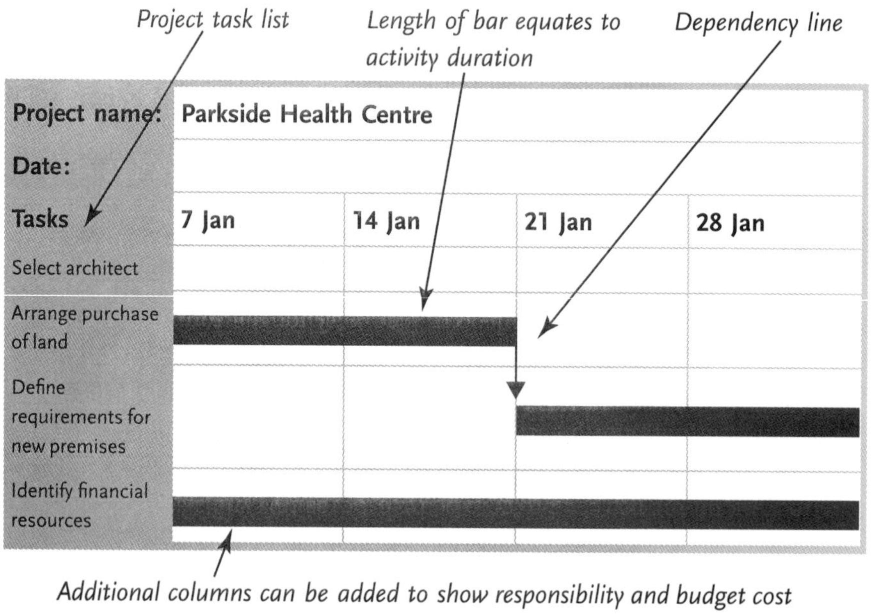

Additional columns can be added to show responsibility and budget cost

Implementation

At last, some action! During implementation it is wise to identify milestones; points where a significant, measurable event in the project has been completed. These milestones can be recorded on the Gantt chart. You need to think about how you are going to keep people informed about the progress on your project. It may be helpful if you are reporting at regular intervals to develop a one-page standard template, containing information on the overall progress, completion of milestones, any outstanding problems, costs to date against budget, and the next milestone for completion. Then it's all systems go. If you want have a launch meeting that's fine, but make sure that everyone knows it's happening.

Managing a budget

In Primary Care, many changes at practice level are never formally costed or resourced. A major factor in failing to complete projects is that adequate people resources at the right level and with the right amount of skills have not been freed up to work on the project. So try to be realistic, as this will also reduce the risk of not delivering within budget.

Smaller projects may not present any real challenge, but for larger, more complex ones it will be more difficult both to build and manage the budget. To build the budget, each task within the project needs to be examined in terms of equipment, materials, training, and labour. The total for the complete project will then be reached. Most projects within Primary Care will not need to take into account indirect costs; e.g. costs of office space, access to computers. If setting the budget is proving difficult, why not ask for help from someone who has completed a similar project? An experienced manager may be a great help at this stage.

Managing the budget will be context specific and the method of tracking the budget will depend on what accounting systems are already in place in the organisation. You need to be aware of expenditure that has not yet gone through the accounts so that you are aware of real-time account status. The mechanism for accessing project funds will need to be agreed, as well as procedures in case things do not go to plan. There also needs to be an effective system for recording costs and monitoring the budget. This could be recorded in a simple spreadsheet document that can be kept up to date.

Monitoring and control

Control of the project environment involves three operating modes:
1. Measuring–determining progress by formal and informal reporting.
2. Evaluating–determining cause of deviations from the plan.
3. Correcting–taking actions to correct.

In a smaller project it is no less important to monitor progress. It may be that you just check on your schedule and Gantt chart at regular intervals and if there are problems, modify subsequent plans accordingly. No matter how small the project, though, documenting progress is important and this can be a simple regular entry into a project log.

Projects often change during their lifecycle, some due to events outside your control. The ability to manage these changes is vital to successful project management.

> *A large inner-city practice needs to recruit a new practice manager.*

There are huge challenges that can lie within this simple sounding task, not least arriving at a common understanding of what the practice needs and agreeing the selection process. The overall project goal is clear and it will be simple to know when the project has delivered, because a new practice manager will have been appointed. Identification of who will lead this project is key and this needs to be agreed by all relevant stakeholders, mindful of the skills that this project requires. Resources will need to be found, such as protected time for the project manager and money for advertising, etc. A project plan needs to be written and task list drawn up. The benefit of doing this is everyone knows what is going to happen and when. The implementation phase will then start. Keeping people abreast with progress will be important as will key dates such as closing dates for applications. Risks include no-one applying or finding your selection process doesn't work. Once you have found your new manager and successfully appointed, the project just needs winding up. This doesn't need a report, but keeping the documentation will help with subsequent appointments as will any lessons learnt – both what worked well and what you will do differently next time.

Closing a project

By definition, a project has an end. Closing a project properly is important, not least so that everyone knows that you have arrived there. At this stage something new should exist that did not exist before and there are a number of tasks that may be necessary, such as to:
- meet with the team to acknowledge achievement of project goals
- write a brief final report
- transfer any ongoing responsibilities
- release resources – desk space, computers, etc
- complete final accounts
- celebrate.

The final evaluation

After the project has ended there is still the evaluation to be done. This is an appraisal of how things have gone, what has worked well, and what could have been better. Depending on the size of the project, there may be three tasks at this stage: project assessment, a final written report, and review of personal and team members' performances. The final report should contain:
- an overview of the project, including any revisions to the original project plan

- a summary of major achievements
- an analysis of achievements compared to project goals
- the final accounts for the project
- an evaluation of the organisation of the project
- a description of issues for further investigation
- recommendations for future projects
- any acknowledgements.

Further reading
All projects are unique but there is a wealth of helpful information on project management in books and on the internet that is easy to find, including many ready-made tools and templates.

Frame JD. *The New Project Management.* San Francisco: Jossey-Bass, 1994.

Lockyer K. *Critical Path Analysis and Other Project Network Techniques.* London: Pitman, 1984.

Rosenau MD. *Successful Project Management.* New York: Van Nostrand Reinhold, 1991.

Young TL. *The Handbook of Project Management.* [Revised edn.] London: Kogan Page, 1998.

Chapter 16

From Policy to Practice:
Strategic Planning in Primary Care

Clare Gerada

 KEY MESSAGES

- Involve staff 'on the ground' early to achieve success later.
- First determine whether change is both necessary and desired.
- Clarify the work and the work plan.
- Identify all relevant issues: national, regional, local.
- Gather information.
- Develop a vision.
- Collaborate widely and work in partnership.

Information

Increasingly, GPs and other Primary Care professionals are asked their views on strategic development: how services can be improved, what changes are needed to meet a particular demand, and how to set up a new service from scratch.

General practitioners in particular are aptly placed to offer strategic advice, being locality-based practitioners often serving the same local community for decades. A caseload of around 100 patients each week, across physical, social, and psychological domains, means quite literally, that GPs have their finger on the public's health. Arguably then, GPs can identify problems and solutions more often, and earlier, than any health care manager, an issue that was touched on in Chapter 1. From fundholding to Primary Care Trusts (PCTs), GPs have been the vanguard of developments, chairing meetings, leading on programmes and reviews, and defining the 'vision' of their Primary Care organisation. At the practice level too, GPs are now called upon to make more strategic decisions than their predecessors. Whereas the only difficult issues facing GPs of old was whether or not to buy into new premises or employ a new partner, GPs now have to deal with major public health issues: where to invest resources, how to improve access, and so on. And in today's NHS, GPs across the country are having to wrestle with such strategic issues as whether to enter or leave Personal Medical Service (PMS) pilots, whether to withdraw from out of hours provision, what nationally enhanced services they can provide, and what the skill-mix of their practice should look like? Their decisions now affect not only their own practice but also the health of their local community.

Strategic planning in Primary Care

The degree of engagement with strategy that individual clinicians choose to take up will vary, from participation in partnerships to contributing to national policies. At whatever level the practitioner works, it is vital that they understand the influence they can have in strategic planning and have some understanding of the basic strategic building blocks, such as needs-assessment, consultation, and an action plan for implementation of a strategic vision.

Strategy in context – policy vs. strategy

At the time of writing the NHS is yet again going through enormous change. New initiatives continue to bombard the clinician and have done so now for over a decade. GP Fundholding has come and gone, perhaps to return in the guise of new PMS pilots. GP commissioning groups have been superseded by Primary Care Groups and they in turn by PCTs – these perhaps to mutate into 'Care Trusts'. General Medical Services (GMS) contracts were abandoned in droves in inner-city areas to be replaced by PMS,[1] subsequently PMS Plus, and now we all face the new GMS contract[2] with its challenges, new decisions to be made, and new battlegrounds to be fought over.

In addition to the organisational changes, Primary Care has had to contend with and understand the new Choice Agenda, Out of Hours Review, Access issues, Skill-Mix, and so on. No sooner does a word or agenda become understood than it is succeeded by another, more exciting, newer, better initiative. Anyone working on the front line of Primary Care development, politics, or

---

Box 16.1 **Quangos and acronyms in the NHS.**

NICE	National Institute for Clinical Excellence
NPSA	National Patient Safety Authority
CGST	Clinical Governance Support Team
CHAI	Commission for HealthCare Audit and Inspection
NCAA	National Clinical Assessment Association
CPPIH	Commission for Patient and Public Involvement in Health
LDP	Local Development Plan
SHA	Strategic Health Authority
NES	National Enhanced Scheme
LES	Local Enhanced Schemes
NSF	National Service Framework

service improvement must keep a watchful eye on government dictums and professional thinking, as well as having a passing knowledge of the role of national quangos and three-lettered acronyms (see Box 16.1).

It is vital that the local strategist has an understanding of national policies that underpin local developments – not least because money will not be granted for implementation if the local strategy is at odds with government policy.

At national level, a strategy is set within an overall policy framework, which sets out the key underpinning principals and priorities. For the NHS these objectives were defined in 2000 in *The NHS Plan*,[3] which explained how they would be delivered by sustained increases in funding (see Box 16.2). The purpose and vision of *The NHS Plan* is to give the people of Britain a health service fit for the 21st century, a health service designed and engineered around the patient.

Box 16.2 The key points of *The NHS Plan* relevant to Primary Care.

- 500 one-stop health centres by 2004
- 3000 surgeries upgraded by 2004
- 2000 more GPs and 450 more registrars by 2004
- NHS Lift, a new private–public partnership, to develop premises
- 1000 specialist GPs
- Annual appraisal

The health and social care priorities that underpin *The NHS Plan* and by definition the NHS are as follows:

- Improving access to all services through:
  - Better emergency care
  - Reduced waiting, increased booking for appointments and admission, and more choice for patients
- Focusing on improving services and outcomes in:
  - Cancer
  - Coronary heart disease
  - Mental health
  - Older people
  - Improving life chances for children
- Improving the overall experience of patients
- Reducing health inequalities
- Contributing to the cross-governmental drive to reduce drug misuse

Shifting the Balance of Power[4] is the programme of change brought about to empower frontline staff and patients in the NHS. It is part of the implementation of *The NHS Plan*. The main feature of change has been giving locally based PCTs the role of running the NHS and improving health in their areas. This has meant abolishing existing Health Authorities and creating new ones that serve larger areas and have a more strategic role. The Department of Health is also refocusing to reflect these changes, including the abolition of its regional offices.

Strategic planning – a framework

For any GP or fellow professional leading strategic development, whether at practice, PCT, or Strategic Health Authority level, it is important to understand the process and the impact that implementing the strategy may have. The next section of this chapter provides a framework for strategic planning and drawing up a business, or strategic, plan.

Strategic planning defines the vision; project planning (see Chapter 15) defines the activities needed to implement that vision. GPs are likely to be involved in both processes, by first being part of the process of planning and then by supporting the implementation.

Phase 1

Getting ready – clarifying the work and work plan. Embarking on strategic change is not a single-minded exercise, performed in isolation, perhaps by the senior partner and the practice manager or the PCT Chief Executive; instead, and to use the jargon, it must have stakeholder involvement and commitment. To prepare itself, however, an organisation must first address whether change is necessary and secondly, that it is ready to change. Essentially, this comes down to whether the leaders of the organisation are truly committed to the effort and can devote the necessary attention to looking at the big picture. Change is always difficult and full of risks that cannot ever be fully predicted. Change creates work, not just for the strategist but also for all the clinicians, managers, and administrative staff that have to implement the new strategy. Change is always resisted and uncomfortable and only by strong leadership can it be accomplished. At practice level this leadership may come from a partner or practice manager – with the others enthused and willing to follow. The larger the organisation, the greater the difficulty in enthusing others who may not see any immediate benefit for themselves (see Chapter 8, 'Managing Change Effectively').

Stakeholder analysis is a simple technique that may be useful in defining commitment and the level of 'buy in' necessary for a plan to succeed. At this stage of proceedings, this will help you focus your persuasive energies most productively.

Try this at home

Stakeholder analysis

- Think of something that you would like to implement: a reorganisation, a new service, a practice improvement.
- List the individuals or groups that have an interest in your plan.
- Across the top draw three columns: 'Opposed', 'Neutral', 'Supportive'.
- Indicate with an 'x' where each stakeholder is at the moment.
- Draw an arrow moving the 'x' to the column that that individual would have to be in for your plan to succeed.
- It may be enough just to shift some stakeholders to neutral but essential to obtain the active support of others.

An organisation that sees itself ready for change must then perform tasks to pave the way for the change process:

- Identify specific issues or choices that the planning process should address (key local and national strategies, plans and targets).
- Clarify roles (who does what in the process).
- Create a planning/key stakeholder group.
- Identify the decisions that need to be made and information that needs to be collected to help make them.

Phase 2

Information gathering. All good plans are based on solid information and common agreement as to the starting point of the planning activity.

An important part of strategic planning, thinking, and management is an awareness of resources and where the change may lead, bearing in mind the continually evolving environment. Assessing the current situation and placing it into some sort of future context means obtaining up-to-date information about strengths, weaknesses, and performance. This information will highlight the critical issues that the organisation faces and that its strategic plan must address. These could include a variety of concerns, such as funding, workforce issues, political imperatives, changing regulations, changing emphasis (patients, access, choice), changing population and demographics, and so on. These critical issues will help to organise and sketch the strategic plan.

This phase of strategic planning will yield a database of important information – current access times, skill-mix, waiting times for services, and so on – depending on the specific area under scrutiny.

Phase 3

Developing the vision. This phase involves outlining the organisation's general strategic direction – its long-term goals and specific objectives – in terms of *mission* and *vision*.

A *mission* statement typically describes an organisation in terms of its purpose (why it exists, what it seeks to accomplish), its core activity (e.g. primary health care provision), and its values (principals or beliefs that guide the members). In contrast, a *vision* statement presents an image of what successful change will look like; for example, 'All patients will have access to their GP within 48 hours or less'.

Phase 4

Working in partnership. Partnership working is an important part of strategic development and a central plank of government policy. Successful partnerships require tangible outcomes and positive engagement of all the partners, be they in health or social care domains. There must be a clear, shared vision of what is required and well-defined roles and responsibilities, respect for cultural and professional differences, and an agreed procedure for setting priorities.

Phase 5

Implementation. Perhaps the hardest part of any strategy is its implementation. All too often the designers of the strategy have no first-hand knowledge of implementation at frontline level and ideas and objectives on paper become impossible to implement in the real, busy, tense life of Primary Care. Involving GPs and colleagues from other Primary Care professions at all levels of strategic development reduces the risks and improves the chances of implementation.

Putting a business plan together

A strategic or business plan is a document summarising the future direction of your organisation over a given time period. It highlights those areas of development that the organisation believes to be of importance and is, effectively, the commitment of your strategic plan to paper. In Primary Care, the process of drawing up a business plan can be usefully considered in the following six steps. These steps are illustrated with a practical case study based around the issue of drugs misuse. Readers working in other fields, medical education for instance, will be able to apply this model to their own operational environment.

Six steps to a Primary Care business plan

1. Identify the national and local priorities and the key targets for delivery over the next (say) three years.
2. Agree the capacity needed to deliver them.
3. Determine the specific responsibilities of each health and social care organisation.
4. Create robust plans based on the involvement of staff and the public that show systematically how improvements will be made.
5. Establish sound local arrangements for monitoring progress and NHS performance management that link into national arrangements.
6. Improve communication and accountability to the public locally so as to demonstrate progress and the value added year on year.

Step One: *Identify the national and local priorities and the key targets for delivery over the next (say) three years.*

- *Drugs strategy*
- *Models of Care[5]*
- *NHS Plan*
- *Local policies around managing drug users*

Step Two: *Agree the capacity needed to deliver them.*

Identify existing providers of community/Primary Care shared care drug services, from mental health trusts, Primary Care (GPs with special clinical interest, nurse prescribers, nurse specialists), voluntary sector, and other (e.g. private) sectors.

Identify potential providers of Primary Care/shared care. At this stage it may be possible to identify key GPs who may be interested in undertaking training to a higher level.

Identify practices able and willing to provide national enhanced services and map these across the geographical area to ensure sufficient capacity across the PCT.

Map gaps in provision of shared care using PCT boundaries as a guide.

Where are services currently, who provides, where are the gaps, what is the level of current interest amongst GPs? What about GPs and nurses with special clinical interests? Is there a move to create nationally enhanced services for drug users?

Step Three: *Determine the specific responsibilities of each health and social care organisation.*

This should reflect the national policy documents, which define the type of services that should be provided within a local health economy, the treatment domains, and commissioning framework. So for example, Models of Care define four levels of service provision. Tier 1 includes non-substance misuse specific services requiring integration with drug and alcohol treatment, such as housing, health promotion, etc; Tier 2 includes Open Access Drug and Alcohol Services; Tier 3 includes structured community-based services; Tier 4 includes residential services.

Step Four: *Create robust plans based on the involvement of staff and the public that show systematically how improvements will be made.*

This can be based on the number of clinicians involved in treatment, the number of patients seen, patient surveys of care, or more formal audits.

Step Five: *Establish sound local arrangements for monitoring progress and NHS performance management that link into national arrangements.*

This may be from numbers of patients in treatment, number of GPs actively involved in the care of drug users, numbers notified, etc.

Step Six: *Improve communication and accountability to the public locally so as to demonstrate progress and the value added year on year.*

References

1. Lewis RM, Gillam S (eds.) *Transforming Primary Care: personal medical services in the new NHS*. London: King's Fund, 1999.
2. British Medical Association. *New GMS Contract 2003*. London: BMA, 2003.
3. Secretary of State for Health. *The NHS Plan: a plan for investment, a plan for reform*. [Cm 4818–1.] London: The Stationery Office, 2000.
4. NHS Executive. *Shifting the Balance of Power*. Leeds: NHSE, 2001.
5. National Treatment Agency for Substance Misuse. *Models of Care for Treatment of Adult Drug Misusers: framework for developing local systems of effective drug misuse treatment in England*. London: National Treatment Agency, 2002.

Chapter 17

Leadership

Neil Jackson

Those who win one hundred triumphs in one hundred conflicts do not have supreme skill. Those who have supreme skill use strategy to bend others without coming to conflict.

Sun Tzu

 KEY MESSAGES

- Leadership is concerned with achieving results through people.
- Effective leadership is characterised by intelligence, credibility, humanity, courage, and discipline.
- In a learning organisation leaders are designers, stewards, and teachers.
- Strategic leadership must encompass task, team, and the individual.
- Leadership style is best defined according to the needs of the followers.
- Reform and investment in the new National Health Service will be achieved through a new generation of managerial and clinical leaders.
- Effective leaders must show some personal qualities but also team- and organisation-centred competencies.

Introduction

Leadership is concerned with achieving results through people and historically has been placed in the context of warfare. More recently, leadership has been identified as an important function within the wider spectrum of management and the concept has been welcomed enthusiastically throughout business, industry, and the public sector. The term *strategic leadership* has also become fashionable, but here again is an implied reference to the military model as illustrated by the following dictionary definition of strategy:

strategy n. *the art or science of the planning or conduct of a war.*[1]

This chapter on leadership is divided into four sections:
1. Leadership – an historical perspective.
2. Strategic leadership – modern concepts.
3. Strategic leadership in the NHS.
4. Effective leadership in Primary Care.

Leadership through the ages – three role models

The hero

Throughout the centuries, men and women have emerged as leaders for many different or circumstantial reasons, and often at times of crisis, democratic election, or by dint of birthright. What is a leader and how does he or she exemplify leadership? Many of us when asked to bring a prominent leader to mind would evoke an image of a romantic hero, perhaps blessed with striking physical attributes, who is charismatic and capable of influencing and inspiring large numbers of people to follow or to fight 'the good cause'. Such an individual might also command total respect and unquestioning loyalty from his or her band of followers. The 'Warrior King' Richard Cœur-de-Lion (1157–99) was one such romantic hero, renowned for his exploits as a crusading knight and accomplished warlord. It is said that he achieved fame at home and abroad both as a chivalrous knight and a brilliant but cautious general. In terms of leadership he combined both the inspiration to energise the troops around him with the ability to set strategic direction, make appropriate decisions, and to plan warfare in great detail.

It might also be argued that Richard Cœur-de-Lion was an exemplar of 'knowledge in leadership', whereby in any given situation a man or woman who knows what to do and how to do it is willingly obeyed and followed by other people.

The strategist

Some fifteen centuries before Richard's crusade, the great military hero Sun Tzu wrote the *Art of War*,[2] a magnificent military treatise in which he embodied the core principles for achieving success over all opposing forces. In his treatise, Sun Tzu described the five fundamentals of strategy that act as the great work of the organisation:
1. Tao – inspiring people to share in the same ideals and expectations, sharing in life and death.
2. Nature – the dark or light, the cold or hot, the systems of time.
3. Situation – the distant or immediate, the obstructed or easy, the broad or narrow, the chances of life or death.

4. Leadership – intelligence, credibility, humanity, courage, and discipline.

5. Art – a flexible system wherein the 'master' or 'sovereign' and its officials employ the Tao.

Here there is an emphasis not just on leadership alone but on strategy. Sun Tzu further emphasised the need for leaders to be familiar with all five fundamentals, because the triumphant would be those who understood them, and the defeated would be those who did not.

The facilitator

Contrast the above with a definition of leadership coined in more recent times. Senge[3] places his leader at the developmental heart of the *learning organisation*:

> *In a learning organisation, leaders are designers, stewards and teachers. They are responsible for building organisations where people continually expand their capabilities to understand complexity, clarify vision and improve shared mental models – that is they are responsible for learning.*

Leadership – modern concepts

Primary Care Trusts (PCTs) are relatively new NHS organisations responsible for commissioning and providing appropriate local health care in partnership with local authorities, especially social services, and with other relevant agencies. As such, PCTs are at the centre of the government's plans for investment and reform in the new NHS. The role and function of PCTs extends to assessing the health needs of their local community and reducing health inequalities, whilst also planning for health improvement and delivering wider objectives for social and economic regeneration through local partnerships. In addition, PCTs have responsibility for the management, integration, and development of Primary Care services; i.e. medical, dental, optical, and pharmaceutical.

PCTs must also take responsibility for clinical governance, which includes setting standards for the provision of primary care; monitoring standards of care; dealing with poor performance; and professional development and support.

All this is a tall order to deliver and presents considerable challenges for each PCT. One of the keys to success is strategic leadership throughout the PCT organisation from Chief Executive level downwards. This is in keeping with The NHS Plan's emphasis on developing leadership across and throughout the NHS.

Strategic leadership

Strategic leadership has been succinctly described by Adair,[3] who describes a 'three-circle' model that encompasses three broad functions of leadership relating to the **task**, the **team**, and the **individual** (see Figure 17.1).

Figure 17.1 **Strategic leadership**

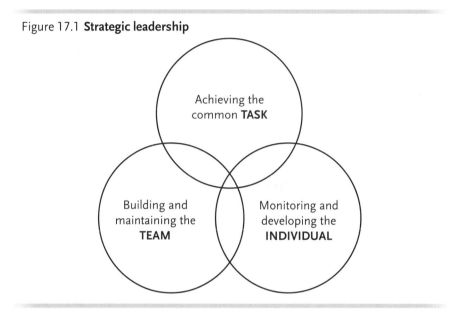

Adair enlarges on this model and defines a number of leadership tasks (see Box 17.1).

Box 17.1 **The tasks of leadership.**

Defining the task	What are the purpose, aims, and objectives? Why is the work worthwhile?
Planning	How you are going to get from where you are now to where you want to be?
Briefing	The ability to communicate; getting across to people the task and the plan.
Controlling	Making sure that all resources and energies are properly harnessed.
Supporting	Setting and maintaining organisational and team values and standards.
Informing	Bringing information to the group and from the group – the linking function of leadership.
Reviewing	Establishing and applying the success criteria appropriate to the field.

Adair goes on to emphasise the distributed nature of leadership; that is, it is disseminated throughout an organisation, not just located at the top, and that it operates at three broad levels: *team, operational,* and *strategic.*

Team. The leader of 10–20 people with clearly specified tasks to achieve.

Operational. The leader of one of the main parts of the organisation and more than one team leader under his/her control (a leader of leaders).

Strategic. The leader of the whole organisation, with a number of operational leaders under his/her personal direction.

Leadership styles

Much has been previously written about leadership styles. Pettinger[5] describes three kinds of style commonly exhibited by leaders:
1. Autocratic (benevolent or tyrannical).
2. Consultative.
3. Democratic.

Thus, at one end of the spectrum an authoritarian approach exists where the leader makes all the final decisions; in the middle of the spectrum a participative approach is utilised where the leader makes decisions after consultation with the group members; and at the other end of the spectrum decisions are made collectively by the group, if necessary by voting.

More recent research into the behaviours of over 30,000 executives by the consulting firm Hay/McBer[6] expanded this taxonomy, defining six distinct leadership styles: coercive, authorative, affiliative, democratic, pacesetting, and coaching. Hay/McBer further discovered that successful executives were adept at switching between styles, depending on the climate or situation.

Situational leadership

Hersey and Blanchard[7,8] have previously advanced the theory of situational leadership, which proposes that the right leadership style needs to be selected based on the needs of followers, and this in turn will ensure successful leadership. Here the emphasis on the followers in leadership effectiveness reflects the fact that it is the followers who ultimately accept or reject the leader, whose effectiveness is dependent upon their actions or inactions.

Situational leadership is considered by Hersey and Blanchard as a model consisting of two main components based around task and relationship behaviours; i.e. *specific leadership behaviours* and *follower readiness.* These are described as follows:

Specific leadership behaviours
- *Telling* (high task–low relationship). The leader defines roles and tells people what, how, when, and where to do various tasks. It emphasises directive behaviour.
- *Selling* (high task–high relationship). The leader provides both directive behaviour and supportive behaviour.
- *Participating* (low task–high relationship). The leader and follower share in decision making, with the main role of the leader being facilitating and communicating.
- *Delegating* (low task–low relationship). The leader provides little direction or support.

Follower readiness. Four stages of readiness are defined:
1. **R1** People are both unable and either unwilling or too insecure to take responsibility to do something. They are neither competent nor confident.
2. **R2** People are unable but willing to do the necessary job tasks. They are motivated but currently lack the appropriate skills.
3. **R3** People are able but unwilling or too apprehensive to do what the leader wants.
4. **R4** People are both able and willing to do what is asked of them.

Within the situational leadership model the two components are integrated and it is postulated that as followers reach high levels of readiness or maturity, the leader responds by decreasing control over activities and also decreasing relationship behaviour as well. Thus the importance of followers is recognised and any limitations in their ability and motivation can be compensated for by their leaders.

Strategic leadership in the NHS

The *NHS Plan*[9] heralded far-reaching changes across the NHS with a comprehensive programme of reform and investment to promote a health service fit for the 21st century. The plan also lays heavy emphasis on leadership in the NHS with the development of a new generation of managerial and clinical leaders. The NHS Modernisation Agency[10] was founded in April 2001 to modernise services and to develop leadership in the NHS, through a leadership centre.

The role of leaders in the NHS, as defined in government health policy and promoted through the leadership centre, is to:
- improve patient care, treatment, and experience
- promote a healthier population
- enhance the NHS's reputation as a well-managed and accountable organisation
- motivate and develop staff.

The NHS Leadership Qualities Framework[11] has recently been introduced, which defines key characteristics, attitudes, and behaviours that are required for leaders in the NHS to deliver *The NHS Plan*. A total of 15 characteristics or qualities are defined within the framework arranged under three group headings: personal qualities, setting direction, and delivering the service. It is hoped that the framework will encourage NHS leaders to become more creative and receptive to change, with a focus on accountability and an emphasis on working through teams and networks in the NHS.

Effective leadership in Primary Care

So far we have defined leadership in terms of the virtue of an individual, the strategic tasks needed to be undertaken, and the leadership style adopted. As you will have realised by now, there are many ways of looking at the elusive concept of effective leadership. As a medical educationalist, I make no apologies for a final model, that of key competencies.

The list that follows is based on my considerable experience of observing Postgraduate Deans, Directors of Postgraduate General Practice Education, and other health care professionals with leadership roles in the service and education and training systems of the NHS. Although these areas of competency will be considered in the context of Primary Care, they are generic and apply to leadership in both the public and private sector or business management domains.

Key competencies for effective leadership
Personal qualities
- Good listener and communicator
- Self-awareness
- Self-confidence
- Well-developed interpersonal skills
- Well-developed sense of strategic vision
- Knowing when to follow rather than lead
- Fair, open, and honest
- Commitment and sense of purpose
- Consistency of behaviour
- Problem-solving skills
- Decision-making skills
- Accountable
- Business-management skills (managing limited resources)
- Appropriate personal and professional values
- Negotiator and mediator (ability to influence when necessary)
- Life-long learner

Team-centred

- A good role model
- Enables delivery on imperatives and facilitating scope for creativity and innovation
- Ensures a balance between tasks and team members
- Promotes an evidence-based approach to work
- Team-building skills (taking into account the strengths and weaknesses of each team member)
- Promotes a corporate approach by the team in line with the stated aspirations of the whole organisation
- Enables team members to reach their full potential
- Fosters a culture of life-long learning and reflective practice
- Recognises the need to take some risks and accept some mistakes

Organisation-centred

- Ability to work in whole systems but to focus-down where appropriate (macro to micro working)
- Ability to work across the four dimensions of policy, strategy, operational, and team
- Works in collaborative partnership with other organisations
- Maintains a balance between local and national priorities
- Builds a shared vision at all levels in the organisation
- Promotes the concept of a learning organisation

A successful application was made by an Associate Director in my own organisation, the London Deanery, to the Department of Health (DH) for funding to support a clinical experience scheme for refugee doctors. The scheme is designed as an essential part of a whole education and training pathway for refugee doctors from the point of entry in the UK to becoming a GP, and is one of a raft of local GP recruitment and retention initiatives.

The tasks of the Associate Director were wide ranging: setting up a Steering Group comprised of a number of collaborative organisations to oversee the whole project; appointing and developing a team including a course organiser and other support workers to run the scheme; developing a critical mass of practices to support refugee doctors during their Primary Care attachment; establishing appropriate deanery recruitment procedures for entry by refugee doctors into the scheme; establishing a database for all refugee doctors on the scheme; project evaluation and drafting progress reports for the DH; and finally making the case for recurring funding having pump-primed the whole initiative from the DH funding originally secured.

In this example, not only the personal qualities and team-centred attributes of leadership are highlighted, but also the organisation-centred attributes that are crucial to the success of the initiative.

Conclusion

Leadership will remain a key challenge for the future in the NHS and indeed for any other public sector service and the private sector. In addition to leading from the front, Chief Executives and senior managers must have well-developed technical and professional competence in their field of practice. At the same time they must ensure a creative and participative culture in their teams and organisations and fully share in the risks, challenges, and performance of their workforce. There is also an ultimate responsibility to ensure the right focus on the needs of patients and carers by ensuring the development of a workforce that is 'fit for purpose'. NHS leaders must also take some responsibility for developing the leadership ability and capacity across all disciplines in teams and organisations within the NHS.

Try this at home

Think of a leader you admire.
- What qualities does he/she exhibit?

Think of a leader who has failed or been replaced.
- What were the reasons for this?

Think of a situation in which you were called upon to be a leader.
- What leadership style did you use?
- Was it the most appropriate for the situation?
- How do you know?

References

1. *Collins English Dictionary.* London: Collins, 1979.
2. Wing RL. *The Art of Strategy: the leading modern translation of Sun Tzu's classic the Art of War.* London: Thorsons, 1997.
3. Senge PM. *The Fifth Disciple: the art and practice of the learning organisation.* London: Century Business, 1992.
4. Adair J. *Effective Strategic Leadership.* London: MacMillian, 2002.
5. Pettinger R. *Introduction to Management.* [2nd edn.] London: MacMillan, 1997.

6.   Goleman D. Leadership that gets results. *Harvard Business Review* 2000; March-April.

7.   Hersey P, Blanchard KH. 'So you want to know your leadership style?' *Training and Development Journal* 1974; Feb: 1–15.

8.   Hersey P, Blanchard KH. *Management of Organisational Behaviour: utilising human resources.* [6th edn.] Englewood Cliffs, NJ: Prentice Hall, 1993.

9.   Secretary of State for Health. *The NHS Plan – a plan for investment, a plan for reform.* London: Department of Health, 2000.

10. The NHS Modernisation Agency: www.modernnhs.nhs.uk.

11. The NHS Leadership Qualities Framework: www.nhsleadershipqualities.nhs.uk.

Writers and thinkers referred to in the text

Nigel Edwards is currently the Policy Director of the NHS Confederation, the membership organisation that represents all Strategic Health Authorities and over 90% of Trusts and Primary Care Trusts in the UK. His job is to influence health policy on behalf of the member organisations and help focus dialogue with the government. Edwards is also a visiting Professor to the London School of Hygiene and Tropical Medicine.

Donald M Berwick is President and Chief Executive Office of the USA's Institute for Healthcare Improvement, a non-profit organisation dedicated to improving the quality of health care systems through education, research, and demonstration projects, and through fostering collaboration among health care organisations and their leaders. Berwick has written widely on health care policy, decision analysis, technology assessment, and health care quality management.

Professor Ian Kennedy, chairman of the Bristol Inquiry, is the shadow chair of CHAI, the new Commission for Health Audit and Inspection. Currently Professor of Health Law, Ethics and Policy at University College, London, he is a former president of the Centre of Medical Law and Ethics (which he founded in 1978), member of the Medicines Commission, and the Department of Health's Expert Advisory Group on Aids. He has chaired the Secretary of State for Health's Advisory Group on Xenotransplantation and the Minister of Agriculture's Advisory Group on Quarantine.

Max Weber (1864–1920) was both an economist and one of the founding fathers of sociology. In his most famous book, *The Protestant Ethic and the Spirit of Capitalism,* he found the seeds of capitalism in the Protestant work ethic. In *Politics as a Vocation,* which he wrote in 1919, Weber defined a taxonomy of authority, or 'legitimations of domination'; means by which men, or the state, might have authority over others. These he classified as traditional, rational/ legal, and charismatic.

Peter F Drucker is a writer, teacher, and consultant specialising in strategy and policy for businesses and social sector organisations. He has worked with many of the world's largest corporations as well as with non-profit organisations, small and entrepreneurial companies, and with the governments of the USA, Canada, Japan, and Mexico. Drucker is the author of 31 books, 15 of which are on management. One of the world's experts on the contemporary organisation, *Business Week* has called him 'the most enduring management thinker of our time'.

Peter Senge studied how firms and organisations develop adaptive capabilities for many years at the Massachusetts Institute of Technology, but it was his 1990 book, *The Fifth Discipline*, that finally brought him deserved recognition. He now spends a considerable amount of time lecturing, and working with, managers and executives in companies, not-for-profit organisations, schools, and government organisations all over the world.

Abraham Maslow (1908–1970). Born in New York, the son of uneducated Russian émigrés, Malsow rose to prominence with his theories of personality development. Maslow's hierarchy of needs was an alternative to the depressing determinism of Freud and Skinner. He felt that people are basically trustworthy, self-protecting, and self-governing and that humans tend toward growth and love provided lower order needs are satisfied. Maslow was an inspirational figure for the humanistic psychology movement and his book, *Motivation and Personality* became a cornerstone of motivational theory.

Bruce Tuckman published his *Forming, Storming, Norming, Performing* model of group relations in 1965 and added a fifth stage, *Adjourning*, in the 1970s. Tuckman's theory remains a good explanation of team development and behaviour. Dr Tuckman is currently Professor in Philosophical, Psychological, and Comparative Studies at Ohio State University with an interest in motivation, procrastination, and self-regulatory behaviour.

Meredith Belbin developed his now world-famous team roles out of research conducted at the Henley Management College. *Management Teams – Why they succeed or fail* has since been cited by the *Financial Times* as one of the top 50 business books of all time. Belbin has had an illustrious career and following some years as a management consultant he went on to become Chairman of the Industrial Training Research Unit and Director of the Employment Development Unit at Cambridge University, and Senior Associate of the Institute of Management Studies.

Katharine Cook Briggs (1875–1968) and her daughter **Isabel Briggs Myers** (1897–1980) developed their theory of personality type based on the work of Carl Jung. Inspired by the waste of human potential during World War II, with the realisation that there was an acute need for a wider understanding of human differences, it was Isabel that was responsible for the design of the Myers–Briggs Type Indicator (MBTI) instrument. The MBTI has gone on to become the most widely used and highly respected personality inventory of all time. It is taken by at 2–3 million people each year and has been translated into sixteen languages.

David Clarence McClelland (1938–98) taught and lectured as an academic on the east coast of the United States throughout his career studying motivation and the achievement need. McClelland pioneered workplace motivational thinking, developing achievement-based motivational theory and models. He was a strong advocate of the supremacy of competency-based testing over IQ and personality tests. His ideas, closely related to the motivational theories of Frederick Herzberg, have since been widely adopted in many organisations. McClelland is most noted for describing three types of motivational need, which he identified in his 1988 book, *Human Motivation*: achievement motivation (n-ach), authority/power motivation (n-pow), and affiliation motivation (n-affil).

Neil Rackham is now chairman of a highly successful research consultancy firm in the USA. Much of his work stems from research he conducted while a postgraduate research fellow at Sheffield, where he developed a range of behaviour analysis techniques that allow precise statistical measurement of interactive skills. Rackham has since used these research tools to study areas such as selling and negotiating where success depends on complex interpersonal skills.

Charles Handy has at one time or another been a broadcaster, oil executive, economist, management consultant, and Chairman of the Royal Society of Arts. Handy has had a huge influence on the way we view the organisations in which we work. While Professor there, Handy developed the London Business School's first MBA and his book, *Understanding Organisations* remains a core text for all students of management theory.

Alvin Toffler is the author, and co-author, of a number of influential books about change, the future, and how to cope with it. He has written about society, culture, the media, organisations, science, computers, politics, and economics. His three best known publications are: *The Third Wave, Future Shock*, and *Powershift*.

John Harvey-Jones earned his status as a business 'guru' from his work at ICI where, after only 30 months as Chairman, he had turned the loss-making company into a highly profitable organisation. A believer in informality, collective leadership and a high level of conflict, his sometimes strident public profile and flamboyant management style has attracted considerable attention. Harvey-Jones has since been the Chancellor of Bradford University, a Vice President of the Royal Society of Arts, Vice Chairman of the Policy Studies Institute and the Institute of Marketing, and a Trustee of the Science

Museum. He is probably best known for his two BBC Television Series, *Troubleshooter* filmed in 1986, and in 1990.

Chris Argyris for over 50 years – first as a faculty member of Yale University and latterly at Harvard – has been one of the foremost thinkers in the fields of organisational learning and development. The concept of single loop and double loop learning that he developed with Donald Schön has been his most influential model, but Argyris has also researched and written widely on the impact of formal organisational structures, control systems, and management on individuals, organisational change, and the extent to which human reasoning, as opposed to behaviour, can become the basis for diagnosis and action.

Donald Alan Schön (1930–1997) trained as a philosopher, but it was his concern with the development of reflective practice and learning systems within organisations and communities for which he is remembered. An interest in the improvisation and structures of jazz was mirrored in his academic writing, most notably in his exploration of professionals' ability to receive information about and respond to the surrounding environment. Three elements of his thinking are particularly noteworthy: learning systems (and learning societies and institutions); double-loop and organisational learning (arising out of his collaboration with Chris Argyris); and the relationship of reflection-in-action to professional activity.

Rosabeth Moss Kanter is the Professor of Business Administration at Harvard Business School and former editor of the *Harvard Business Review*. She is an internationally known business leader, a consultant to major corporations around the world, award-winning author, and expert on strategy, innovation, and the management of change. Named as one of the 50 most powerful women in the world by *The Times*, Moss Kanter has received 19 honorary doctoral degrees and over a dozen leadership awards. She has served on many corporate boards and is a Fellow of the World Economic Forum.

Kurt Lewin (1890–1947) was one of the most charismatic psychologists of his generation and the father of modern social psychology. Lewin's training in psychology began in 1910 in Berlin and he continued working there until 1932 when he emigrated to America working as an academic first in Iowa and then at the Massachusetts Institute of Technology where he established the Research Center for Group Dynamics. Lewin is most renowned for his development of the *field theory*, the idea that human behaviour is the function of both the person and the environment; i.e. that one's behaviour is related both to personal characteristics and to the social situation in which one finds oneself. Lewin's work lead to the development of actual field research on human behaviour. A hugely important legacy, as his approach has guided experiments in the field of social cognition, social motivation, and group processes ever since.

Stephen R Covey is best known for his book *The Seven Habits of Highly Effective People*, which has sold over 10 million copies worldwide. He is an internationally respected authority on leadership and organisational effectiveness. *Time* magazine has hailed Covey as one of the 25 most influential Americans.

Henry Mintzberg is the Cleghorn Professor of Management Studies at McGill University in Montreal. His academic work spans several decades over which Mintzberg has shifted his focus from identifying what it is that managers actually do (*The Nature of Managerial Work*, 1973), to the structure of organisations (*Structure in Fives: developing effective organisations*, 1983), the development of a theoretical basis to strategy (*Strategy Safari*, 1998) and most recently, transforming management education (*Developing Managers, Not MBAs*, in press).

Paul Hersey and **Kenneth Blanchard** developed a model of situational leadership in the 1970s, which was later popularised through the *One Minute Manager* series. They suggested that the leadership style should be adapted to the maturity of the followers, that is their confidence in performing the task, and their level of skill. This lead to a four-part taxonomy of leadership styles: telling, selling, participating, delegating. Their best selling book (now in its 8th edition) *Management of Organizational Behavior: leading human resources* succinctly summarises much of the organisational theory found in the chapter on leadership.

Daniel Goleman is a psychologist who for many years reported on the brain and behavioural sciences for *The New York Times*. Following the publication of his 1995 book, *Emotional Intelligence*, Goleman now consults internationally and lectures on the world stage. Goleman argues that human competencies like self-awareness, self-discipline, persistence, and empathy are of greater consequence than IQ in much of life, that we ignore the decline in these competencies at our peril. Perhaps more scarily for parents, he argues that children can – and should – be taught these abilities.

David W Keirsey is a clinical psychologist who worked for public schools for 20 years as a corrective interventionist, and followed this with 11 years training therapists and pathologists, at California State University, in the art of changing dysfunctional behaviour in children and adults. Keirsey and Bates's *Please Understand Me*, first published in 1978, sold nearly 2 million copies in its first 20 years, becoming a perennial best seller all over the world. The book became a favourite training and counselling guide in many institutions helping people find their personality style. Kiersey's four temperaments are rooted in the work of Isabel Briggs Myers and can be explored further at: www.keirsey.com/matrix.html.

John Adair is internationally acknowledged as having had a significant influence on leadership and management development in both the business and military spheres. He has seen military service, lectured at Sandhurst, worked extensively as a consultant, held professorships in Leadership Studies, and authored well-received leadership and management books. More than one million managers throughout the world went through the Action-Centred Leadership course that he pioneered in the 1970s.

Index